T0259530

Nutrition

Editor

JÖRG MAYER

VETERINARY CLINICS
OF NORTH AMERICA:
EXOTIC ANIMAL PRACTICE

www.vetexotic.theclinics.com

Consulting Editor
AGNES E. RUPLEY

September 2014 • Volume 17 • Number 3

ELSEVIER

1600 John F. Kennedy Boulevard • Suite 1800 • Philadelphia, Pennsylvania, 19103-2899
http://www.vetexotic.theclinics.com

**VETERINARY CLINICS OF NORTH AMERICA: EXOTIC ANIMAL PRACTICE Volume 17, Number 3
September 2014 ISSN 1094-9194, ISBN-13: 978-0-323-32349-9**

Editor: Patrick Manley
Developmental Editor: Casey Jackson

Veterinary Clinics of North America: Exotic Animal Practice (ISSN 1094-9194) is published in January, May, and September by Elsevier, Inc., 360 Park Avenue South, New York, NY 10010-1710. Subscription prices are $255.00 per year for US individuals, $399.00 per year for US institutions, $130.00 per year for US students and residents, $305.00 per year for Canadian individuals, $482.00 per year for Canadian institutions, $340.00 per year for international individuals, $482.00 per year for international institutions and $165.00 per year for Canadian and foreign students/ residents. To receive student/resident rate, orders must be accompanied by name of affiliated institution, date of term, and the *signature* of program/residency coordinator on institution letterhead. Orders will be billed at individual rate until proof of status is received. Foreign air speed delivery is included in all *Clinics* subscription prices. All prices are subject to change without notice. **POSTMASTER:** Send address changes to *Veterinary Clinics of North America: Exotic Animal Practice*, Elsevier Health Sciences Division, Subscription Customer Service, 3251 Riverport Lane, Maryland Heights, MO 63043. **Customer Service: Telephone: 1-800-654-2452** (U.S. and Canada); **1-314-447-8871** (outside U.S. and Canada). **Fax: 1-314-447-8029. E-mail: journalscustomerservice-usa@elsevier.com** (for print support); **journalsonlinesupport-usa@elsevier.com** (for online support).

Reprints. For copies of 100 or more of articles in this publication, please contact the Commercial Reprints Department, Elsevier Inc., 360 Park Avenue South, New York, New York 10010-1710. Tel.: 212-633-3874; Fax: 212-633-3820; E-mail: reprints@elsevier.com.

Veterinary Clinics of North America: Exotic Animal Practice is covered in *MEDLINE/PubMed (Index Medicus)*.

Contributors

CONSULTING EDITOR

AGNES E. RUPLEY, DVM
Diplomate, American Board of Veterinary Practitioners–Avian Practice; Director and Chief Veterinarian, All Pets Medical & Laser Surgical Center, College Station, Texas

EDITOR

JÖRG MAYER, DVM, MSc
Diplomate American Board of Veterinary Practitioners (ECM); Diplomate European College of Zoological Medicine (Small mammal); Department of Small Animal Medicine and Surgery, College of Veterinary Medicine, Associate Professor of Zoological Medicine, University of Georgia, Athens, Georgia

AUTHORS

JANA BRAUN, DVM
VCA Silver Lake Animal Hospital, Everett, Washington

LEIGH ANN CLAYTON, DVM
Diplomate American Board of Veterinary Practitioners (Avian, Reptile/Amphibian); Director, Animal Health National Aquarium, Baltimore, Maryland

CARMEN M.H. COLITZ, DVM, PhD
Diplomate American College of Veterinary Ophthalmologists; Animal Necessity, LLC, New York, New York and All Animal Eye Care, Inc., Jupiter, Florida

MIKE CORCORAN, DVM, CertAqV
Associate Veterinarian, Arizona Exotic Animal Hospital, Mesa, Arizona; Founding Member, American Association of Fish Veterinarians, Allentown, Pennsylvania; Secretary, World Aquatic Veterinary Medical Association, Stafford, United Kingdom

KERRIN GRANT, MS
Wildlife Care Director and Nutritionist, ICU, The Wildlife Center, Espanola, New Mexico

CATHY A. JOHNSON-DELANEY, BS, DVM
Washington Ferret Rescue and Shelter, Kirkland, Washington

LA'TOYA LATNEY, DVM, Post-Doc, MSCE
Chief of Service and Attending Clinician, Exotic Companion Animal Medicine and Surgery, University of Pennsylvania Veterinary Teaching Hospital, Philadelphia, Pennsylvania

CHRISTOPH MANS, DVM
Special Species Health Service, Department of Surgical Sciences, School of Veterinary Medicine, University of Wisconsin, Madison, Wisconsin

JÖRG MAYER, DVM, MSc
Diplomate American Board of Veterinary Practitioners (ECM); Diplomate European
College of Zoological Medicine (Small mammal); Department of Small Animal Medicine
and Surgery, College of Veterinary Medicine, Associate Professor of Zoological Medicine,
University of Georgia, Athens, Georgia

JOHANNA MEJIA-FAVA, DVM, PhD,
Animal Necessity, LLC, New York, New York

SUSAN E. OROSZ, PhD, DVM
Diplomate American Board of Veterinary Practitioners (Avian); DECZM (Avian); Bird and
Exotic Pet Wellness Center, Toledo, Ohio

LAILA MAFTOUM PROENÇA, MV, DVM, MS, PhD
Department of Small Animal Medicine and Surgery, College of Veterinary Medicine,
University of Georgia, Athens, Georgia

HELEN ROBERTS-SWEENEY, DVM
Aquatic Veterinary Services of WNY, Williamsville, New York; Founding Member,
American Association of Fish Veterinarians, Allentown, Pennsylvania

Contents

Fish are the most popular pets in the United States based on numbers and high-quality medical care is coming to be expected by owners. Increasing numbers of veterinarians are responding to this need and providing veterinary care for aquatic animals. Part of good medical care for exotic animals is advice on husbandry, including nutrition. However, there are numerous missing areas of research for the nutritional needs of many ornamental fish species. What is known for food species can be combined with what is known for ornamental species to give nutritional advice to owners to maximize health in these animals.

The study of amphibian nutrition requires a detailed review of species-specific natural prey analysis. Invertebrate nutrient composition has been formally studied for more than 60 years and presents the following conclusions: (1) in general, insects are poor in overall calcium content; (2) larval insects have high fat and protein components; and (3) altering the gut contents of some insects can improve their overall nutritive quality. The fat-soluble vitamin profile for most inverts is lacking. There are new guidelines for calcium and vitamin A supplementation that can help augment invertebrate nutrient profiles to match the minimum NRC requirements established for rats.

Nutritional disorders of captive reptiles remain very common despite the increasing knowledge about reptile husbandry and nutrition. Many nutritional disorders are diagnosed late in the disease process; often secondary complications, such as pathologic fractures in reptiles suffering from nutritional secondary hyperparathyroidism have occurred. Therefore, every attempt should be made to educate reptile owners and keepers about the proper care and dietary needs of reptiles under their care because all nutritional disorders seen in captive reptiles are preventable.

Psittacine birds eat plant-based foods. Birds in the wild seem to be able to balance their energy needs, amino acids, and calcium. Companion birds in captivity do not do as well when self-selecting, and balanced diets are needed to improve their general health. A nutritional history is important to determine whether the avian patient is in balance nutritionally. Understanding the various sources of the fat-soluble vitamins, calcium, and protein will help guide clients to provide nutritious foods for their birds. Owners need to learn to use foraging as a major source of their bird's diet and techniques.

Marsupials comprise an interesting group of mammals, which are increasingly being kept as pets. Few actual feeding trials have been published, although many anecdotal diets have years of usage with good success. Marsupials have dental and digestive tract adaptations that allow them to use specific niches in their environments. Knowing the diet in the wild is instrumental in designing diets used in captivity.

The domestic ferret (*Mustela putorious furo*) is a strict carnivore, also referred to as an obligate carnivore. Its dentition and gastrointestinal tract are adapted to a carnivorous diet. Its ancestor, the European polecat (*Mustela putorius*), feeds on birds and other small vertebrates. Domesticated ferrets have been fed mink feeds, cat foods, and now mostly subsist on commercial ferret diets formulated specifically to meet their needs.

This article summarizes the literature regarding digestive strategies and captive diets of common rodent pocket pets. A comparison is made between the 2 suborders in which chinchillas, guinea pigs, hamsters, and gerbils occur, highlighting digestive anatomy and dietary adaptations. Recommended captive diets are provided, as well as common nutritionally related health issues that may be presented to veterinary clinics.

Dietary management can be used with drug therapy for the successful treatment of many diseases. Therapeutic nutrition is well-recognized in dogs and cats and is beginning to increase among other pet species, including rabbits. The nutritional component of some rabbit diseases (eg, urolithiasis) is not completely understood, and the clinician should evaluate the use of prescription diets based on the scientific literature and individual needs. Long-term feeding trials are needed to further evaluate the efficacy of prescription diets in rabbits. Prescription diets are available for selected diseases in rabbits, including diets for immediate-term, short-term, and long-term management.

Johanna Mejia-Fava and Carmen M.H. Colitz

The use of supplements has become commonplace in an effort to complement traditional therapy and as part of long-term preventive health plans. This article discusses historical and present uses of antioxidants, vitamins, and herbs. By complementing traditional medicine with holistic and alternative nutrition and supplements, the overall health and wellness of exotic pets can be enhanced and balanced. Further research is needed for understanding the strengths and uses of supplements in exotic species. Going back to the animals' origin and roots bring clinicians closer to nature and its healing powers.

VETERINARY CLINICS OF NORTH AMERICA: EXOTIC ANIMAL PRACTICE

THE CLINICS ARE NOW AVAILABLE ONLINE!
Access your subscription at:
www.theclinics.com

Preface

On the Importance of Putting the Right Fuel into the Engine

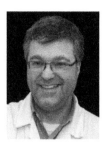

Jörg Mayer, DVM, MSc, DABVP (ECM),
DECZM (small mammal)
Editor

Every engine needs a specific kind of fuel to operate at an optimal level. Exactly the same is true in biology. The different species of animals need their specialized fuel to function well. Nearly every day you can read some new story on how important certain foods are for human health or how poor food is linked to various diseases or pathologies. We are just in the beginning of translating this knowledge to our patients. I personally find animal nutrition one of the most interesting but also one of the most challenging topics in veterinary medicine. When asked to be an editor for an issue of the series, it was an easy choice for me to pick Nutrition as the topic. I was also pleased to see that the May 2014 issue of the series was on Gasteroenterology, which make a perfect couple.

I am very excited about this issue in your hands (or on your screen), as I was able to recruit excellent authors to bring you up-to-date and clinically important information. I truly feel blessed to be working with such great colleagues, who love to share their knowledge and expertise with us. One of the great aspects of exotic animal medicine is the constant growth of new information, which has the potential to truly impact the well-being of many generations of exotic pets. We are also currently experiencing an exciting era in the pet food industry as more and more companies are catering to our requests to offer specialty foods for our exotic pets. While we are still far behind regarding the situation when compared with products offered for domesticated pets, the gap is being slowly but surely closed, as every year more specialty nutrition products are being offered. I am convinced that the current issue of the series offers important and significant information on a vast variety of topics regarding nutrition.

I hope that you will find this issue an exciting read, and hopefully the authors are able to encourage all of us to continue to keep nutrition on our daily radar and also to be able to communicate the importance to the owners of these exotic pets as they have the power to prevent many diseases with the right nutrition. I clearly learned a lot about

Vet Clin Exot Anim 17 (2014) ix–x
http://dx.doi.org/10.1016/j.cvex.2014.06.001
1094-9194/14/$ – see front matter © 2014 Elsevier Inc. All rights reserved.

nutrition during the editing process and I hope that I can pass this important information on to the owners and to directly implement this in my daily clinical routine. I would like to take the opportunity to thank all the authors who contributed to this issue as they clearly took a large amount of time out of their busy schedules to make us all better veterinarians, help our patients, and thereby look great to others! Imagine me singing an emotional version of Wayne Newton's "Danke schön" here!

Jörg Mayer, DVM, MSc, DABVP (ECM), DECZM (small mammal)
Zoological Medicine
University of Georgia
College of Veterinary Medicine
501 D. W. Brooks Drive
Athens, GA 30602, USA

E-mail address:
mayerj@uga.edu

Aquatic Animal Nutrition for the Exotic Animal Practitioner

Mike Corcoran, DVM, CertAqV[a,b,c,*], Helen Roberts-Sweeney, DVM[b,d]

KEYWORDS

- Fish nutrition • Fish medicine • Aquatic animal diets • Koi nutrition
- Tropical fish nutrition • Aquarium nutrition

KEY POINTS

- Fish have higher protein requirements and lower carbohydrate requirements than most other exotic animals.
- There are essential amino acids and vitamin requirements that must be addressed by diet.
- Omega-3 fatty acids are required by aquatic species.
- Essential amino acids and omega-3 fatty acids are best provided by fish meal protein in the diet.
- Most minerals can be obtained from the water.
- Fish have lower basal energy requirements than land animals because of their ability to excrete ammonia without first forming uric acid or urea.
- Nutritional needs are variable for many species depending on temperature, season, age, day length, and other external cues.
- In addition to the proper food, behavioral needs must be addressed for proper nutrition.
- Improper nutrition leads to health problems similar to many other species.

NUTRIENT REQUIREMENTS FOR FOOD SELECTION

Proteins

Proteins in fish, just like other animals, are the building blocks of the body. They are used to form muscle, skin, and other tissues. They are essential for immune function, catalyzing reactions, and replicating DNA. They are also used for energy. In fish, proteins are more important than carbohydrates as an energy source. Part of the reason is

Disclosures: There are no conflicts of interest to report.
[a] Arizona Exotic Animal Hospital, 744 North Center Street, Suite 101, Mesa, AZ 85201, USA;
[b] American Association of Fish Veterinarians, 4580 Crackersport Road, Allentown, PA 18104, USA; [c] World Aquatic Veterinary Medical Association, 132 Lichfield Road, Stafford, Staffordshire ST17 4LE, United Kingdom; [d] Aquatic Veterinary Services of WNY, Williamsville, NY 14221, USA
* Corresponding author. Arizona Exotic Animal Hospital, 744 North Center Street, Suite 101, Mesa, AZ 85201.
E-mail address: mcorcoran@azeah.com

that fish have lower energy requirements than mammals.[1] There are also significant differences in carbohydrate metabolism in fish that are discussed further later.

As a percentage basis in the diet, there is some dispute in the research. The percentage based on studies varies from 25% to 55% of the diet.[1–6] The low end of this range is based on the need to use the minimal protein amount in production fish in order to save money. The best consensus is a range of 35% to 45% for herbivorous and omnivorous fish, and 40% to 55% for carnivorous fish.[2–4] These percentages are general guidelines and depend on many other factors. The percentage of proteins needs to be balanced as a percentage of the total dietary energy because fish eat only enough to meet dietary energy requirements. Proteins in excess of this need could lead to deficiency in one or more of the other nutrients.[3,4]

The quality of protein is as important, or more important, than the amount. The protein must be bioavailable and provide all essential amino acids. Essential amino acids are those that are unable to be produced by the organism from other constituents.

Research on several different species of fish has identified the same 10 essential amino acids, which are similar to those for many other species of animals.[1,2,4,6–9] Among the essential amino acids, arginine seems to be one of the most important to consider in supplementation (**Box 1**). Fish seem to have a greater need for arginine than do mammals.[1,2,8] In mammals, the urea cycle can act as a source for arginine, but fish lack this ability.[2] As a percentage of the total protein in the diet, the essential amino acids should compose 50% to 60%.[2,5,7] This amount helps prevent deficiency in amino acids when fish eat to their total energy requirements.

The best source of protein is animal protein. Fish meal provides the best choice for the source of essential amino acids and digestibility of proteins.[3,6,7,10] If greater than 50% of the protein is plant protein there can be decreased complement activity in the immune system.[6] Sometimes availability and cost require that a mixture of fish protein and other protein sources be used. Alternative protein sources should first be other animal proteins. If vegetable proteins are used, soybean meal is the best source.[1,2]

Fat

Fats in the diet provide a valuable energy source. Fats are also deposited in the body to provide thermal insulation from the surrounding environment of an organism. In fish,

---

Box 1
Essential amino acids in aquatic animals

1. Arginine
2. Histidine
3. Isoleucine
4. Leucine
5. Lysine
6. Methionine
7. Phenylalanine
8. Threonine
9. Tryptophan
10. Valine

Data from Refs.[1,2,4,9]

fats are deposited in a way that helps to streamline the body and reduce resistance in the water when swimming. In addition, fats are precursor molecules for many hormones and sterols such as cholesterol, estrogen, and testosterone.

Fats should constitute 15% to 25% of the diet.[4,9] Unlike mammals, fish have a specific requirement for n-3 fatty acids. All fish have a requirement for 18:2 and 18:3 n-3 fatty acids, in which the numbers indicate fatty acids with a chain 18 units long with 2 or 3 double bonds, respectively.[1,2,4,7] There is also evidence that marine fish are unable to lengthen the chains of fatty acids, which leads to requirements for 20:5 and 22:6 n-3 fatty acids in their diets.[4,7]

Fish oils are the best source for all of these requirements. Vegetable oils, with few exceptions, are poor sources of n-3 fatty acids.[7,10] Other animal fats and oils have higher degrees of n-6 fatty acids. Increased n-6 fatty acids can contribute to cardiologic or inflammatory diseases.[7]

Aside from proteins, fats are the most important energy source for most fish. In periods of food deprivation, lipids were the most important energy sources for most fish species.[11] As with other species, excess fats can cause obesity in fish, which is becoming one of the most common preventable diseases in fish.[3]

Carbohydrates

In most species, carbohydrates are a primary energy source in the diet. Blood glucose levels are generally tightly controlled in a narrow range by insulin and other hormones. In fish, the control of blood glucose is less evident. Plasma glucose values are highly variable between species and even within species depending on life stage, feed intake, temperature, and other variables.[11] Various studies have shown fish to be insulin resistant.[6,11] In some studies, after injection of dextrose, fish took more than 24 hours to return to normal blood sugar levels.

The levels returned to normal faster in omnivorous fish than in carnivorous fish.[11] During times of decreasing temperature, omnivorous fish tend to store more glycogen in the liver. This glycogen was depleted during a time of food deprivation in fasting carp in one study.[12] There is also some indication that melatonin affects the uptake of carbohydrates in preparation for a period of food deprivation in response to shortened day length.[11]

Most carbohydrates are poorly digested by fish, with a digestibility of 20% to 40% in most species.[2] Carbohydrates in the form of starches are more digestible. Increased dietary starch content yielded higher levels of glycogen in the liver, and this glycogen was used during food deprivation in an omnivorous fish.[4,11] Several studies indicate that 10% of the diet as starch is the optimal level.[7,11] The total carbohydrates in the diet for omnivorous fish should be 25% to 40% and less than 20% for carnivores.[4] Higher glucose levels affect liver function.[7,11]

Vitamins

A variety of studies have assessed the vitamin requirements of different fish. Although the studies are mainly performed on production fish, similar needs were found in diverse species, and results were similar to many land animals.[4,7] These findings have been used to support the ability to generalize for ornamental species until further studies are conducted on these species; however, caution should be used in this interpretation, especially with fat-soluble vitamins. Further studies should be conducted on common ornamental species to determine vitamin requirements in the diets.

The studies conducted to date indicate that most water-soluble vitamins and several fat-soluble vitamins should be supplemented. It seems that vitamins A, C, D, E, and K are all likely to require supplementation in fish diets.[6,13]

Vitamin A deficiency has been shown to cause skeletal deformity in fish. Larvae deprived of vitamin A developed lordosis, kyphosis, scoliosis, retarded growth, and impairment of bone and cartilage metabolism.[13] Excesses of vitamin A were also implicated in the deformities through compression and fusion of vertebrae.[13]

Vitamins C and E have been found to help the immune response in fish.[1,7] Daily requirements of vitamin C have been found to be 25 to 50 mg/kg of feed in several different species of fish. Ten times the daily dose of vitamin C has also been found to be safe and to help the function of the immune system.[1,9,14]

One of the biggest concerns with vitamins is stability in the food. Vitamins are made labile by temperature changes, moisture, and exposure to light. Water-soluble vitamins may also leach from food items in less than 1 minute when put in the water for feeding.[3,7] Vitamin stability is the limiting factor in the storage time for food. Vitamin C is one of the most labile and stabilized vitamin C (L-ascorbyl-2-polyphosphate) should be used. Even with stabilized vitamin C, the storage time for food should be no longer than 90 days.[3,9]

Minerals

Minerals are stable natural elements that are required by the organism for normal function. Some examples are sodium, potassium, magnesium, calcium, and phosphorus. For most elements required by fish, there is little need for supplementation in the diet. Most minerals required by fish are obtained easily from the water.[1,4,6,7] Even fresh water of moderate hardness has been shown to provide adequate calcium for fish to compensate for dietary inadequacies.[4]

The only mineral that has been identified in fish that must be supplemented in the diet is phosphorus. Phosphorus is generally found in water in concentrations that are too low to meet the needs of the fish without dietary supplementation.[1,4,5,7] Because many fish do not have a true stomach, the phosphorus in fish diets must be highly soluble to be absorbed well by some species.[1] Forms such as phylate are biologically unavailable to fish.[5] As a percentage of the diet, 0.3% phosphorus is recommended.[5]

In order for this advice to be supported, the practitioner must ensure that water quality is adequate. For trace elements to be absorbed in adequate amounts to meet the requirements of the fish they must be present in the water. A freshwater system using reverse osmosis water of low hardness may not meet the needs of the fish without the addition of aquarium salts, trace elements, and/or calcium. Infrequent water changes can also lead to depletion of trace elements in fresh or salt water. The frequency of water changes needed to avoid this problem depends on many factors including the size of the system, number of animals in the system, hardness of the water, and pH. The best way to manage important trace elements in water is to test levels weekly to biweekly.

Some trace elements can also be harmful in levels not much higher than those necessary to meet the needs of the animals. Copper is a good example. Copper is required for red blood cell production and for the health of the immune system; however, there are some species of fish that cannot tolerate copper levels of 0.15 ppm in the water even for short periods of time. Chronic toxicity can occur with less than 10% of that concentration.[15] Invertebrates, elasmobranchs, and copper-sensitive fish have issues with toxicity at far lower levels.[16–18] In addition to copper, zinc, nickel, and several other minerals have a low therapeutic index. Detailed information on mineral toxicity is outside the scope of this article.

Probiotics

With the continuing awareness of the overuse of antibiotics in medicine, clients are becoming more interested in the potential benefits of probiotics. With evidence-based medicine, practitioners must strive to make recommendations based on research and empirical evidence. There is some good proof that some probiotics not only are safe but that they help digestion and help reduce disease. In order to be effective, bacteria used in probiotics must tolerate bile and the acidity of the stomach to enter the intestinal tract. They must also adhere to the intestine and must effectively compete against pathogenic bacteria. Lactic acid bacteria have been tested for these parameters. *Lactococcus lactis*, *Lactobacillus plantarum*, and *Lactobacillus fermentum* all tolerated oral administration and effectively adhered to intestinal mucosa. When challenged with pathogenic bacteria, all strains effectively competed and reduced mortality.[19] Another study tested levels of a commercial prebiotic added to a basal diet. Common carp fed the diet with 1.5 g/kg of the commercial prebiotic had reduced mortality when challenged with *Aeromonas hydrophila* infection.[20]

Color Enhancers

One unique aspect of nutrition with aquatic animals is the addition of color enhancers. Many fish species are valued for the coloration of the scales and skin. Pigments involved in coloration include melanin, carotenoids, and guanine. Melanin and guanine can be produced by most fish and do not need to be supplemented in the diet.[6] Carotenoids are used in many feeds to enhance the coloration of fish. Many different carotenoids are offered on the market and clients often have questions regarding recommendations. Choices include synthetic materials, yeasts, bacteria, and fungi. One study compared 2 algae (*Chlorella vulgaris* and *Haematococcus pluvialis*) and 1 cyanobacteria (*Arthrospira maxima*) with a synthetic astaxanthin. They were tested for the results on goldfish and 2 variety of koi. The best results were obtained from the 2 algae, with *C vulgaris* giving the best results.[21] This finding allows a good recommendation for a natural product rather than synthetic products to clients concerned with color enhancement in their fish.

Fiber

Fiber is the material in terrestrial plants that is indigestible to vertebrates. There is little fiber in aquatic plants, and therefore fiber should play a minor role in the diet of aquatic animals (**Box 2**). The fiber content should be less than 5%.[6]

Medicated Feeds

There are many commercially available medicated feeds, and the practitioner should expect some questions regarding their use. Most of the medicated feeds available

---

Box 2
Summary of nutrition requirements

	Herbivore and Omnivore	Carnivore
Protein	35–45%	40–55%
Fat	15–25%	15–25%
Carbohydrate	25–40%	<20%
Fiber	<5%	<5%

Proteins primarily fish meal and other animal protein.
Fats with a significant source of n-3 fatty acids.
Carbohydrates as starch.
Vitamins A, C, D, E, K and B vitamins.
Phosphorus 0.3%.
    Data from Refs.[1–4,6,7,10,11]

were designed for specific needs of commercial food fish production. Those available to pet owners and hobbyists are often not regulated by the US Food and Drug Administration and may have no empirical evidence for their use. In the author's experience, many of the foods contain inappropriate antibiotics; unknown concentrations of medication; or a mixture of antibiotic, antifungal, and antiparasitic medications. The author cautions clients regarding use of these products because of potential development of drug resistance and unnecessary side effects of multiple medications. However, many people see their use as a less expensive alternative to proper diagnosis and treatment based on an accurate working diagnosis, or they use the feeds at the advice of well-intentioned paraprofessionals or retailers.

Summary and Practical Applications

Using this information in a practical situation can be challenging. There are hundreds of commercial foods available, and even more homemade diets. Often the practitioner is asked to evaluate a diet by the client with little time for preparation.

With most commercial foods, only the American Association of Feed Control Officials (AAFCO) minimum information and ingredients list may be available for review. This list allows evaluation of the percentage of protein (should be 30%–50%), crude fat (minimum listed only), crude fiber (should be <5%), and moisture (no set guideline, but may affect interpretation of protein and fat in some foods).

The ingredients list should be evaluated next. In a good-quality food, fish meal or other animal protein should be one of the first ingredients. Little plant protein should be listed. If plant protein is listed, soy is best; other plant proteins should be low on the list of ingredients. Vitamin sources can be identified. The practitioner should look for stabilized vitamin C and a list of other vitamins. A source of digestible phosphate can be identified along with other mineral supplementation. In addition, identify the color enhancers used in the food, if any.

For more detailed evaluation, the manufacturer of the diet normally needs to be contacted. The practitioner should be cautioned that some information may be deemed proprietary by the manufacturer and may not be available for evaluation. If too little information is shared on request, the author generally recommends a different diet. Additional considerations based on common types of fish in the ornamental fish industry are discussed later.

FOOD SELECTION: OTHER CONSIDERATIONS
Energy

Following an understanding of the individual requirements for fish, an understanding of the fundamental differences in the energy requirements of fish helps practitioners guide clients away from some of the most common mistakes related to nutrition. The information presented earlier helps with food selection recommendations, but the biggest nutritional problem for aquatic animals is overfeeding. Owners often have difficulty judging the amount of food to be offered. The typical mammal uses 30% of the energy intake for basal metabolic energy requirements. This figure is only 3% to 5% for fish because fish readily excrete ammonia through the gills and have little need to convert ammonia through the urea cycle for excretion.[1]

Overfeeding contributes to the 2 most common food-related health issues: obesity and poor water quality. Obesity can be addressed best by following the previous recommendations when selecting food. Aquatic animals generally eat to meet their energy requirements. Obesity is likely a sign that the selected food has low dietary energy compared with the level of proteins, lipids, or other essential elements. The excess intake of proteins or lipids in excess of what is required for energy needs is then converted to stored fat.[1,4]

Organic material is naturally converted to ammonia through digestion or decomposition. In most species, ammonia is further converted to urea and sometimes to uric acid. The urea cycle is absent or greatly reduced in fish, and ammonia is effectively removed through the gills into the surrounding water. Overfeeding of protein leads to increased ammonia in the water of the pond or aquarium through excretion of ingested foods or decomposition of uneaten foods.[1,4,6] Ammonia and ammonium are toxic to fish. Biological filtration converts ammonia to nitrites, then to nitrates in a healthy system (**Fig. 1**). Each step is less toxic, and nitrates are either removed through water changes or conversion to nitrogen gas. The efficiency of biological filtration is limited by the size of the system and surface area for the growth of bacteria in the biological filter. Any ammonia in excess of what can be converted will cause health issues with the inhabitants of the system.[1,6,9,14]

Food Formulations

The formulation of the feed has a great deal to do with the acceptance by the animal and the delivery of nutrients in an aquatic environment. Fish diets are available as live foods, liquid food, frozen foods, pellets, and flakes. The formulation must ensure that the nutrients are effectively delivered to the fish and digested properly. There are unique challenges for aquatic animal diets that must be considered.

Most diets do not involve live feeding, but some fish do require live food. In general, larval fish require live food for survival. In one study, fish larvae raised initially on dry food showed 100% mortality by 15 days compared with 100% survival in larvae raised

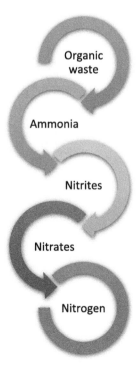

Fig. 1. Ammonia cycle.

on live food up to 15 mg body weight.[22] Live food has the advantage of stimulating natural behavior in fish and may offer enrichment. The drawback is the potential for introduction of parasites or disease. There are also the ethical implications of placing prey in an enclosed space with their predator.

Liquid and frozen diets are similar. Most are prey-based diets containing small crustaceans, eggs, or other prey in a liquid base, often starch based. The liquid may be supplemented with vitamins or minerals. The liquid diets are packaged fresh. Liquid diets have short shelf lives, but can offer good nutritional profiles and a diet that resembles the natural food that fish eat in the wild.[2] Frozen food has a longer shelf life and a reduced chance of introducing disease, but caution must be used regarding the stability of vitamins with freezing.

Pellets and flakes are dry foods. They are the most prevalent commercial diets available to hobbyists. The extrusion process used to make these diets allow feeds to have higher energy content and increases the digestibility of the nutrients. Gelatinization of starch in this process also increases the stability of the diet and availability of vitamins.[4] Vitamins must be added after the heating process to avoid breakdown of vital bonds.[7] Flakes are floating foods that need to be eaten at the surface. Pellets can be either floating or sinking foods depending on the formulation, allowing fast-sinking pellets to be used for bottom-feeding fish and slow-sinking pellets for those that feed in the center of the water column. Pellets are also available in different sizes and shapes (**Fig. 2**).

Storage

Proper storage of any diet is one of the most important considerations to ensure that proper nutrition is delivered to the fish. With regard to storage of food, temperature, humidity, and lighting can all affect the viability of the diet offered. Improper storage of foods with regard to these considerations can lead to decreased nutritional value at best and fatal toxicity at worst.

With prolonged storage, fats and vitamins can oxidize and undergo damaging changes from the oxidation. Polyunsaturated fatty acids, which are present in most fish diets, can oxidize and become rancid, especially if there is inadequate vitamin E

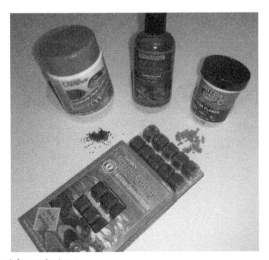

Fig. 2. Various food formulations.

or other antioxidants in the diet. The rancid odor is usually difficult to detect among the normal smells associated with fish meal. Many owners do not detect rancid food until there is loss of numerous fish and other possible causes are exhausted.[3,7] Oxidized fats can form toxic compounds that result in anemia, splenomegaly, ascites, and nephrosis.[3] Many fish are able to detect the tastes of the rancid fatty acids and avoid toxicity from ingestion, but may instead incur nutritional deficiencies or hepatic lipidosis.[4]

Vitamins are also oxidized in storage, particularly the fat-soluble vitamins. Continuing to use feed that has oxidized vitamins can result in health problems secondary to hypovitaminosis. The clinical signs of vitamin deficiencies are often nonspecific and easily confused with other health issues, again making these conditions difficult to detect.[2,3,7] Any animals showing outward signs of illness should have supplemental vitamins offered as part of the treatment plan, particularly vitamins B and C. Requirements for these vitamins are especially profound during periods of stress.[4,7]

Increased humidity during storage can lead to growth of molds on the foods. Molds on food can produce aflatoxins. Many fish can detect oxidation products associated with this and consequently have decreased food intake, resulting in nutritional deficiencies. If the aflatoxins are consumed they can be toxic to the fish.[4] The toxicity of the dose is usually measured in parts per billion. Aflatoxins are usually not detected by smell, therefore food hygiene and storage conditions must be appropriate.

Any consultation involving illness in fish should include a review of food storage in the history. If the current food has been stored for longer than 90 days, it should be replaced.[3] A maximum of 90 days' storage should also be advised to any clients during preventative medicine screenings or on any care sheets published for client information (**Box 3**).

Behavioral Considerations

The nutritional makeup of the food and the form of the food only matter if the food is ingested by the fish. There are many behavioral considerations that factor into acceptance of food items. Some are similar to other species and some are unique to aquatics. A comprehensive evaluation by species is beyond the scope of this article, but it is appropriate to introduce some of the behavioral considerations to help the practitioner in evaluations and to introduce ideas in order to ensure that behavioral concerns are addressed or that the need for further research is not overlooked. The author has divided these considerations into sensory, social, and environmental concerns for ease of summarizing.

Fish have most of the same senses as land animals. Some have excellent senses of taste, olfaction, sight, or hearing. As previously discussed, many fish recognize the taste or smell of oxidized oils and avoid rancid food. It has also been shown that carnivores prefer alkaline or neutral foods, whereas herbivores tend toward acidic foods.[4]

Box 3
Storage of Food

Protect from light

Protect from moisture

Keep between 70–85 F

Use within 90 days

Data from Refs.[2–4,7]

In addition to the normal senses, fish have a lateral line: a sensory organ running the length of the body from rostrum to tail and located roughly parallel to the spine. The lateral line detects low-frequency vibrations and pressure changes. Elasmobranchs have the ampullae of Lorenzini, specialized organs that detect electrical impulses. These senses are key in detecting prey in the wild.[16] Fish rejecting food may respond to foods that are a different color, size, smell, or taste. The feel of the food may also be a factor.[1,4] Eels have been shown to prefer foods with a soft texture.[1]

Social factors are those behavioral patterns that are either innate or responses to other animals in the system that affect how the fish eats. Eels are a good example of this as well. Eels, gobis, and many other fish have innate drives to hide or inhabit closed spaces.[3] In the wild as well as in captivity they roam only a short distance in the open. Sinking food or focused feeding with tongs or droppers may be required for them to get the necessary dietary food intake. Other fish occupy a specific area in the water column: near the surface, near the bottom, or in the middle. Food may need to be delivered into those areas to ensure that adequate nutrition is offered to those fish.[1,4] The caretaker also has to observe closely for submissive fish who may have decreased food intake or delayed eating.[3] Water-soluble vitamins may be lost once in the water for as little as 30 seconds.[3,7] This loss may lead to vitamin deficiency in submissive fish.

Environmental factors that have been found to affect the feeding habits of fish in the wild include temperature, lighting, tides, lunar cycles, depth, and seasons. Many of these factors are limited to wild conditions, but others are possible to duplicate in captivity and can be used to help improve nutrition. Tides likely increase feeding by increasing available food. Likewise, full moons increase ambient light and may increase feeding activity by making prey easier to locate for nocturnal feeders.[4] In captivity, artificial tidal movement is created in some systems and water pumps increase water flow to create circulation patterns in tanks, although these usually benefit filter-feeding invertebrates more than fish. Lighting is something that can be controlled in most systems. Artificial lighting systems are available for indoor aquariums that effectively simulate the spectrum of light to which fish are exposed in natural conditions. Modern lighting systems can be programmed to simulate sunrise and sunset by slowly varying light levels. They can also simulate lunar cycles with low-level lighting that changes on a 28-day cycle. Many can also create simulated storms or cloud cover moving across the aquarium. Seasonality can be simulated by adjusting day length with the programming. Lighting can be used to adjust fish to meal feeding in most cases.[4]

For outdoor fish, natural rhythms affect the fish and the caretaker needs to understand the influences of these processes and adjust accordingly for care. In general, food intake decreases with shortening days and decreasing water temperatures. Food intake increases as the water temperature increases again and the days increase in length.[4] As feed intake decreases, the caretaker should reduce the food offered to avoid water quality problems. Feeding times should be adjusted to allow digestion to be completed at the warmest part of the day.[2,4]

SPECIFIC RECOMMENDATIONS
Koi

Koi are some of the most frequently treated fish in private practice. Many clients with koi participate in wellness programs and are interested in consultations with veterinarians for preventative medicine. Discussions on nutrition are an important part of that care. In addition, considering nutrition during any treatment plan for an unhealthy koi is essential to successful treatment. There has been research in koi nutrition, much of which is discussed earlier.

There are a large number of commercially available koi diets on the market. Evaluating and recommending diets should be done similarly to the summary earlier in this article. The main protein source should be fish meal. Protein, fat, and carbohydrate requirements are similar to other omnivorous fish, although carbohydrate levels may be slightly higher than in diets for other omnivorous fish. As omnivores, koi are more tolerant of carbohydrates and are likely to use the carbohydrates for energy during periods of starvation.[7,11] However, if there are edible plants or algae in the pond, they are likely to get the carbohydrates needed from grazing in the pond.

Koi also have a need for vitamin C. Specific requirements are not known for koi, but other fish have been found to need 25 to 50 mg/kg in feed for routine supplementation.[1,9] This amount is the author's recommendation for feed, again keeping in mind that it should be stabilized vitamin C and that the feed should be stored for no longer than 90 days.[3,9,15] If being treated for injury or illness, additional vitamin C should be supplemented at up to 10 times this level per day.

Koi tend to significantly decrease their energy output and food intake as temperatures decrease in the pond and as the length of days decrease over the winter months. This change is important for reproductive physiology of the fish and helps avoid reproductive diseases. Many hobbyists and food companies recommend transitions to different diets for the winter. The author could find no reliable research to support the need for this change. As energy output decreases, caretakers should be advised to reduce feeding amount and frequency over the winter, but there should be no need to change the diet.

Tropical Aquarium Fish

Most pet ornamental fish are tropical freshwater or saltwater fish. There are hundreds of species of fish represented in the pet trade. There is a lack of information available for many of these species. There is also likely a wide range of needs for these different species. Although there is some information available for the needs of a few species, the needs for all the inhabitants of a specific aquarium are difficult to determine objectively. As such, the recommendations in this area are largely based on generalized nutritional research, the author's experience, and discussions with other practitioners and aquarists. The most important recommendation for caretakers is recognition of the species in the tank as carnivorous, omnivorous, or herbivorous to help in selection of diets.

For tropical freshwater fish, there are a variety of commercial flaked and pelleted foods available on the market. The author generally recommends evaluating these foods according to the information in the summary given earlier. Fish meal as a primary protein source is desirable, along with soy and other vegetable proteins in smaller amounts. A stable source of vitamin C and the availability of B vitamins and vitamins A, E, D, and K should be found in the ingredients. It is also advisable to observe fish in the aquarium during feedings. Not all fish come to the surface to eat floating flakes in a timely manner. If not all are eating flaked food, then sinking pellets should be used: slow-sinking pellets for fish that stay near the middle of the water column and fast-sinking pellets for those that stay near the bottom of the aquarium.

For tropical marine fish, the author often recommends that a variety of foods be rotated. There are several commercial systems designed for this type of feeding. A variety of shrimp, seaweeds, algae, and eggs can be offered on a rotating basis.

The hope with this is that any unknown nutritional deficiencies are avoided by offering a variety of protein sources to the aquarium inhabitants. Again, careful observation during feeding times should be recommended to ensure that all inhabitants have the opportunity to eat food in a timely manner. The same recommendations apply to these diets for vitamin and mineral supplementation.

Marine Invertebrates

Reef aquariums are gaining popularity as they become easier to maintain. Therefore, it is good for the practitioner to have some knowledge of corals and other invertebrates. Extensive coverage is beyond the scope of this article, but the practitioner should be prepared to correct the basic incorrect elements of so-called common knowledge in the hobby. Many sources state that there is no need to feed invertebrates. Many invertebrates maintain themselves by feeding on algae or other plant sources in the system, but this is not universally true. Any crustaceans should be observed closely and supplemental food should be offered at least weekly even if they are eating algae.

Corals obtain energy from a commensurate relationship with the single-celled photosynthetic organisms known as zooxanthellae. Although this relationship provides most of the nutritional requirement of the coral, it depends on a specific intensity and wavelength of light. It also provides full nutrition for few corals. Most need to be fed with plankton or other food sources (**Fig. 3**).[17,18]

Elasmobranchs

Although uncommon in veterinary practice, elasmobranchs (sharks and rays) are sometimes encountered. Two important considerations should be noted. First, B vitamins should be a consideration in the diet because many of the frozen fish used in the diets contain thiaminases that affect thiamin levels in the diet. Second, iodine needs to be supplemented at high levels for most elasmobranchs. Without proper iodine supplementation, elasmobranchs are more prone to goiter.[16] In addition to supplementation of iodine in the diet, the levels in water should be tested. The level of iodine in the water may be more important than that in the diet. A recent study showed that reduction of iodine in the water after the addition of ozonation led to goiter even in sharks that were given iodine supplements in their diets.[23]

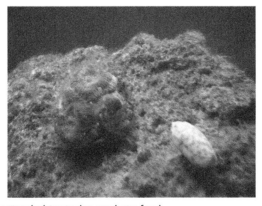

Fig. 3. Coral with extended tentacles ready to feed.

SUMMARY

Nutritional advice is an important part of aquatic animal medicine, just as in any other branch of medicine. There are many areas of fish nutrition that vary greatly from that of other species, and many areas in which research is lacking. As aquatic animals become more popular and more people consider a relationship with a veterinarian to be an important part of the hobby, this research is likely to be completed. The practitioner should keep up with all information available in order to give the best advice possible for their patients.

REFERENCES

1. Lovell RT. Nutrition of aquaculture species. J Anim Sci 1991;69:4193–200.
2. King J. Fish nutrition. Vet Rec 1973;92:546–50.
3. Mayer J. Fish nutrition and related problems. Hartz Exotic Health 2002;1:1–4.
4. Lall SP, Tibbets SM. Nutrition, feeding, and behavior of fish. Vet Clin North Am Exot Anim Pract 2009;12:361–72.
5. Robinson E, Menghe L. A summary of catfish nutrition research. Mississippi State (MS): Mississippi State University; 2005. p. 5–10.
6. Roberts H, editor. Fundamentals of ornamental fish health. Ames (IA): Wiley-Blackwell; 2010. p. 89–101.
7. Olivia-Teles A. Nutrition and health of aquaculture fish. J Fish Dis 2012;35:83–101.
8. Li P, Mai K, Trushenski J, et al. New developments in fish amino acid nutrition: towards functional and environmentally oriented aquafeeds. Amino Acids 2009; 37:43–53.
9. Lewbart GA. Clinical nutrition of ornamental fish. Seminars in Avian and Exotic Pet Medicine 1998;7:154–8.
10. Hardy RW, Gatlin DM, Bureau DP, et al. Nutrient requirements of fish and shrimp: report in brief. Washington, DC: National Academies Press; 2011.
11. Hemre GI, Mommsen TP, Krogdahl A. Carbohydrates in fish nutrition: effects on growth, glucose metabolism and hepatic enzymes. Aquaculture Nutr 2002;8:175–94.
12. Liew HJ, Sinha AK, Mauro N, et al. Fasting goldfish, *Carassius auratus*, and common carp, *Cyprinus carpio*, use different metabolic strategies when swimming. Comp Biochem Physiol A Mol Integr Physiol 2012;163:327–35.
13. Haga Y, Du S, Satoh S, et al. Analysis of the mechanism of skeletal deformity in fish larvae using a vitamin A-induced bone deformity model. Aquaculture 2011; 315:26–33.
14. Fracalossi DM, Allen ME, Nichols DK, et al. Oscars, *Astronotus ocellatus*, have a dietary requirement for vitamin C. J Nutr 1998;128:1745–51.
15. Noga EJ. Fish disease: diagnosis and treatment. 2nd edition. Ames (IA): Wiley-Blackwell; 2010. p. 391–3.
16. Smith M, Warmolts D, Thoney D, et al, editors. Elasmobranch husbandry manual: captive care of sharks, rays and their relatives. Columbus (OH): Ohio Biological Survey; 2004. p. 171, 183–200, 433–40.
17. Borneman E. Aquarium corals: selection, husbandry and natural history. Neptune City (NJ): TFH Publications; 2009. p. 57–69, 343–58.
18. Sprung J, Delbeek C. The reef aquarium: a comprehensive guide to the identification and care of tropical marine invertebrates, vol. 2. Coconut Grove (FL): Ricordea Publishing; 1997. p. 161–4.
19. Balcazar J, Vendrell D, de Blas I, et al. Characterization of probiotic properties of lactic acid bacteria isolated from intestinal microbiota of fish. Aquaculture 2008; 278:188–91.

20. Ebrahimi G, Ouraja H, Sudagar M, et al. Effects of a prebiotic, Immunogen, on feed utilization, body composition, immunity and resistance to *Aeromonas hydrophila* infection in the common carp *Cyprinus carpio* (Linnaeus) fingerlings. J Anim Physiol Anim Nutr 2012;96:591–9.
21. Gouveia L, Rema P, Pereira O, et al. Colouring ornamental fish (*Cyprinus carpio* and *Carassius auratus*) with microalgal biomass. Aquaculture Nutr 2003;9:123–9.
22. Bambroo P. On the diet substitution and adaptation weight in carp *Cyprinus carpio* larvae. Indian J Sci Res 2012;3:133–6.
23. Morris A, Stremme D, Sheppard B, et al. The onset of goiter in several species of sharks following the addition of ozone to a touch pool. J Zoo Wildl Med 2012;43: 621–4.

Updates on Amphibian Nutrition and Nutritive Value of Common Feeder Insects

(●) CrossMark

La'Toya Latney, DVM, Post-Doc, MSCE[a],*,
Leigh Ann Clayton, DVM, DABVP (Avian, Reptile/Amphibian)[b]

KEYWORDS

- Anatomy • Invertebrate prey • Gut-loading • Amphibian • Minerals • Vitamins
- Lipid

KEY POINTS

- The study of amphibian nutrition still requires detailed review of species-specific natural prey analysis.
- Invertebrate nutrient composition has been formally studied for more than 60 years and presents the following conclusions: (1) in general, insects are poor in overall calcium content; (2) larval insects have high fat and protein component; and (3) altering the gut contents of some insects can improve their overall nutritive quality.
- There are new guidelines for calcium and vitamin A supplementation that can help augment invertebrate nutrient profiles to match the minimum National Research Council requirements established for rats.

INTRODUCTION

In comparative medicine, practitioners are commonly faced with clinical manifestations of nutritional imbalances in captive amphibians. Studies that evaluate herptile nutrient minimums, digestion, and prey nutrient bioavailability are scarce.[1,2] Limited data are available for commercially prepared and extruded diets for captive insectivores. Information regarding natural diet of insectivores and insect composition does exist and can be found primarily in comparative physiology journals, zoology-focused and herptile-focused journals such as *Copeia*, *Zoo Biology*, and *Journal of Herpetology*. When comparing species-specific natural diets to commercially available invertebrates, what remain are insects that have poor nutritive value as compared

Disclosures: None.
[a] Exotic Companion Animal Medicine and Surgery, University of Pennsylvania Veterinary Teaching Hospital, 3900 Delancey Street, Office 2107, Philadelphia, PA 19104, USA; [b] Animal Health National Aquarium, 501 Pratt Street, Baltimore, MD 21202, USA
* Corresponding author.
E-mail address: llatney@vet.upenn.edu

with natural diets. In this review, basic amphibian gastrointestinal anatomy and life stage food selection in select species are revisited. A detailed review of the major components of nutrition, insect nutritive value, and common nutritional deficiencies in captive amphibians are provided.

The class Amphibia includes 7000 species that span 3 major orders: Anura (frogs and toads), Caudata (salamanders and newts), and Gymnophiona (caecilians). According to the Amphibian Web database (www.amphibiaweb.org), there are approximately 7258 extant amphibian species as of 2014, which comprise 6398 anura, 660 caudata, and 200 caecilians. A general review of amphibian taxonomy is available for interested readers.[3] This review begins with a review of the larval anurans (tadpoles) and adult gastrointestinal anatomy and natural diet specifications.

AMPHIBIAN GASTROINTESTINAL ANATOMY
Larval Amphibians

With the exception of a few species, most larval anurans have been historically grouped as aquatic, omnivorous, or herbivorous feeders. A classification scheme was developed based on the arrangement of the mouth, operacula, and jaw musculature to identify 5 types of tadpoles based on dietary preference.[4–8] In microphagous, suspension-feeding tadpoles, water is actively siphoned into the oral cavity and directed over filter mucous-covered plates in the pharynx, called the branchial seize.[9,10] This filtering structure can remove bacteria, protozoa, and plankton from the water; however, it can also be used to feed on larger material.[9] The lips are composed of a keratin beak and an oral disc, covered in keratin denticles, surrounding the mouth. The denticles rasp food from vegetation or animal remains, and the branchial sieve siphons the organic debris into the mouth for consumption.[5,9]

As detailed in a previous review, the filtered food is transported by cilia into the esophagus and stomach and peristalsis does not occur.[5,10] The stomach serves as a food storage unit and exists as a small dilatation at the end of the esophagus. Digestion occurs in the elongated and narrow small intestine, which is extensively curled within the coelom.[9,11] The larval stomach widens and lengthens during metamorphosis and extensive glandular development occurs as the midgut shortens and widens in the adult.[9,11]

Larval salamanders and caecilians consume a carnivorous diet as do most adult amphibians; therefore, their gastrointestinal anatomy is similar to that of the adult amphibian. They actively hunt with well-developed jaws to seize prey and peristalsis occurs to move captured prey from the esophagus into the stomach. The stomach contains peptic proteolytic enzymes that begin digestion. During metamorphosis, the cellular composition of the gut changes; however, in general, the larval intestinal tract is grossly similar to that the adult tract.[9,11,12] A review of the complex gastrointestinal changes that occur is available.[13]

Adult Amphibians

The components of the gastrointestinal tract of adult amphibians follow the major anatomic pattern seen comparatively in mammals, with few exceptions. Adult amphibians are carnivorous and their oral cavities are large and wide, which serves to accommodate prey capture.[9] The lips are poorly developed. A choana is present, but forms vary based on species. The teeth assist in capturing prey. Many species secrete mucous from the buccal salivary glands, with the exception of *Pipa*, *Siren*, and *Amphiuma* species. Most species have salivary glands; however, they may be lacking in fully aquatic anurans species.[12] The buccal and salivary glands do not aid in digestion.[10]

Adult amphibians actively hunt and use a specialized tongue to capture and consume invertebrate and vertebrate prey. A detailed review of prey capture mechanisms is available.[8] In general, most terrestrial amphibians possess a mucus-secreting tongue that can extend from the oral cavity and is "flicked out" to capture prey.[6,10,12] Mucous secretions from the tongue, the intermaxillary gland from the roof of the mouth, and muscular contractions of the tongue aid in trapping prey.[10] *Discoglossidae* species have lingual attachments that prevent extension and *Pipa* species have poorly developed tongues.[8–10]

The wide and short esophagus has cilia and mucus-secreting cells that aid in the movement of prey into the stomach. Upper and lower esophageal sphincters are present and esophageal contractions move food boluses into the gut.[9,12] Pepsinogen is produced in the esophagus of *Rana*, *Hyla*, and *Bufo* species; however, the alkaline oral environment prevents activation of the enzyme until it reaches the stomach. Pepsinogen is not produced in the esophagus of *Pipa* species.[9,10]

The stomach, located on the left side on coelom, is composed of a glandular mucosa, submucosa, and tunica musclaris and is the primary location of protein digestion.[9] Hydrochloric acid, produced in the stomach, combines with pepsinogen to form the pepsins that digest protein. Peptic proteolysis and digestion are directly related to ambient temperature and varies among different species.[9] Fundic and pyloric muscular contractions aid in the mechanical breakdown of the food bolus, and a detailed review of motility is available.[9]

Fundic contractions are frequent and serve to move soft, fluid material into the pyloric region. Pyloric contractions are stronger, occur less frequently, and appear to mix food materials as well as move material into the pylorus.[10] Gastric contractions appear to be controlled by the midbrain or medulla and increase in response to increases in ambient temperature.[9] The gastric brooding frog, *Rheobatrachus silus*, ingests fertilized eggs and broods them in the fundus and proximal stomach until the young frogs are fully developed. Gastric acid production is reduced during brooding and its regulation is thought to be controlled by substances produced by the eggs and young.[14]

The pyloric sphincter releases gastric contents into the long small intestinal tract, where most digestion occurs as the ingesta is mixed with pancreatic enzymes and bile, as seen in mammals.[9] Nutrients are actively absorbed within the small intestine and appear to possess fewer folds and villae, which preclude gross identification of specific duodenal, jenjunal, and ileal regions. Cellular composition does vary along the length of the intestine.[9,12,15–18] Seasonal variations in gut size due to volume intake has been demonstrated in adult Andean toad, *Rhinella spinulosa* (formerly *Bufo spinulosus*); however, digestive enzyme activity does not change during periods of food ingestion or during fasting.[19] In this species, Naya and colleagues[19] postulate that the atrophy of digestive organs, particularly the small intestine, is not coupled with the disintegration of villus of the intestinal cells, as has been demonstrated in birds or with the probable decrease of biochemical capacities, as reported in reptiles.

The intestine is highly vascularized and possesses a lymphatic system, and vessels drain the intestines to join the hepatic portal vein as blood is returned to the liver.[10] The gut-associated lymphoid tissue recruits lymphocytes from circulation.[20]

The liver is bilobed in anurans and undivided in urodeles. A gallbladder is present and the biliary system follows mammalian pattern and function, whereby the acidic contents of the intestine stimulate bile release.[10] Amphibian bile improves digestion of fats via the emulsification of digesta into fat particles, forming micelles that are digested by lipase.[9] The pancreas produces insulin, amylase, lipase, and trypsin and is located in the hepatogastric ligament between the duodenum and stomach. The number of pancreatic ducts can vary among species.[9] There is no strong evidence that supports that amphibians can digest keratin, chitin, or cellulose; however, a pancreatic chitinase has been identified in the Japanese Common Toad, *Bufo japonicus*.[21]

The large intestine is the primary location for salt and water resorption and empties fecal material into the cloaca before exiting the body. It usually has a larger diameter than the small intestine and *Rana* species have a valve that separates the small from large intestine.[9,12]

COMPONENTS OF THE AMPHIBIAN DIET

Given the profound diversity of amphibians, it stands to reason that extensive species-specific field research is necessary to analyze the gastrointestinal contents of amphibians to guide captive nutrition guidelines.[22] Captive breeding has provided evidence that some captive diet recommendations have been successful. Most of these diets are based on commercially available invertebrate prey for most adults. There are, however, some unique considerations for specialized larval amphibians.

Specialized Larval Feeders

There are some larval anurans that are well-adapted carnivores, like the Plain's spadefoot toad, *Spea bombifrons*,[23–25] which receives environmental queues after accidental consumption of a tadpole or brine shrimp to engage in cannabalism. Other larval anurans have been classified as opportunistic feeders and undergo resource-based ontogenetic niche shifts.[26,27] In one study that evaluated the feeding ecology of the wood frog, *Lithobates sylvaticus*, leopard frog, *Lithobates pipens*, bullfrog, *Lithobates catesbeinana*, and green frog, *Lithobates clamitans* tadpoles, some degree of carnivory was displayed among all species.[27] Bullfrog tadpoles, and to some degree, closed-canopy wood frog tadpoles, functioned effectively as primary predators in the pond food web. Variable degrees of omnivory were observed, as green frogs consumed more animal matter than leopard frogs and open-canopy wood frogs. This evidence suggests that some can adapt to macrophagous predation and effectively change the dynamics of the pond food web.

Although some larval anurans specialize in carnivory, others species, like the Couch's spadefoot toad, *Scaphiopus couchii*,[28] Amazonian poison frog, *Dendrobates ventrimaculatus*,[29] Strawberry poison dart frog, *Oophaga* (formerly *Dendrobates*) *pumilio*,[30] Eiffinger's tree frog kurixalus, (formerly *Chirixalus*) *eiffingeri*,[31] Vampire flying frog, *Rhacophorus vampyrus*,[32,33] and Mountain chicken frog, *Leptodactylus fallax*,[34] rely on obligatory oophagy. Most studies conclude that this is a specialized feeding strategy designed to eliminate potential resource competitors, increasing resources available for survivors, and providing energy-rich nutrients, which results in an increase in fitness.[28]

Larval tiger salamanders, *Ambystoma tigrinum*, engage in predatory cannabalism when an increase in tadpole population density occurs. Morphologic enlargement of the jaw size of in some normal tadpoles results when crowding occurs and predatory cannabalism is initiated against distantly related tadpoles.[35] In one study, *Ambystoma opacum* preferred to eat sibling tadpoles during cannibalistic feeding as opposed to distantly related individuals.[36]

Some larval caecilian species consume a unique diet item that aids in nutritional support of offspring.[37] The brooding female *Boulengerula taitanus* caecilian undergoes glandular changes within the stratum corneum to provide a rich supply of nutrients for the dermatophagous offspring. Specialized dentition of the young is used to peel and eat the outer layer of their mother's modified skin. Kupfer and colleagues[37] discovered that epidermis of brooding females is up to twice the thickness of that of nonbrooding females, as a result of elongation of the stratified epithelial cells rather than any increase in numbers of cells. Histochemistry reveals that, unlike in non-brooding females, the cytoplasm of modified epidermal cells of brooding females is full of lipid inclusions. A similar finding has been noted in the Neotropical caecilian *Siphonops annulatus*. Fetuses of viviparous caecilians also have a specialized denti-tion[38] that they use to feed on the hypertrophied lining of the maternal oviduct.[39]

INVERTEBRATE COMPOSITION

Invertebrates make up the bulk of the natural diet of most aquatic and terrestrial am-phibians; therefore, a thorough understanding of insect nutrient composition is neces-sary to optimize the nutrition of captive amphibians. Invertebrate composition has been well studied for more than 60 years. The first composition studies were used to evaluate the nutritive quality of mealworm larvae, *Tenebrio molitor*, as a proposed primary diet item for callatrichids,[40] captive pottos, *Perodicticus potto*,[41] tree-shrews, *Tupaia belangeri*,[41] and mouse lemurs, *Microcebus murinus*.[41] Insect culturing proto-cols were subsequently published for the African migratory locust, *Locusta miqratoria*, house cricket, *Acheta domesticus*, waxworm, *Galleria mellonella*, mealworm, *T moli-tor*, and fruit fly, *Drosophilia melanogaster*, which were used as food items for captive insectivores in zoologic gardens.[42] Entomologists have historically studied the nutri-tion of the silkworm, *Bombyx mori*, to optimize feed conversion, larval survival, silk gland health, and cocoon production as a result of a large silk textile industry.[43–45] The black soldier fly larvae, *Hermetia illucens*, or phoenix worm, has been extensively studied as a staple diet for rainbow trout in aquaculture,[46] but has recently become a popular feeder for captive reptiles and amphibians.[1,47]

The following insects have been evaluated for their nutrient composition and **Tables 1** and **2** overview the most current summary of their nutritive profiles.

- Domestic cricket, *A domesticus*[40,48–51]
- Earthworm, *Lumbricus terrestris*[48,52]
- Silkworm, *B mori*[48,53]
- Mealworm larvae and beetles, *T molitor*[40,41,48,52,54–58]
- Fruit flies, *D melanogaster*[42,47,52,58]
- Waxworm, *G mellonella*[48,52,59]
- Superworm larvae and beetle *Zoophobas morio*[48,52,58]
- Termites *Nasutitermes* spp.[60]
- Black soldier fly larvae or phoenix worm, *H illucens*[1,46]
- Madagascar hissing cockroaches, *Gromphadorhina portentosa*[58]
- Butterworm worms, *Chilecomadia moorei*[47]
- Turkistan or red rusty cockroaches, *Blatta Lateralis*[47,58]
- Adult house flies, *Musca domestica*[47]
- Wood louse, *Porcellio scaber*[58]
- False katydid, *Microcentrum rhombifolium*[58]
- Migratory locust, *L migratoria*[42,61]
- Termites, *Nasutitermes* spp.[60]
- Six-spotted cockroach, *Eublaberus distani*[58]
- German cockroach, *Blatella germanica*[62]
- Honey bee, *Apis mellifera*[62]
- Gypsy moth, *Porthetria dispar*[62]
- Slugs, *A subflavus*[62]
- Dung beetle (unknown species)[62]
- Dragonfly nymphs (unknown species)[62]

Table 1
Summary of ME, protein, and fat composition in select insect feeders

	Water (%DM or g/kg)	ME (kcal/kg)	ME (kcal/kg) Energy Density Adjusted	Crude Fat (% DM)	Crude Fat (g/kg)	Crude Protein (%DM)	Crude Protein (g/kg)	Nitrogen (%DM)
Adult house cricket (Finke,[48] 2002)	692 g/kg	1402	4552	22.8[a]	68	64.3[52,a]	205	10.3[52]
Mealworm larvae (Finke,[48] 2002)	619 g/kg	2056	5396	NA	134	51.9[52,a]	187	8.3[52]
Mealworm, adult beetle (Finke,[48] 2002)	637 g/kg	1378	3796	NA	54	NA	237	NA
Mealworm, adult beetle (Oonincx & Dierenfeld,[58] 2012)	61%	NA	NA	17.7	NA	67.65	NA	NA
Superworm larvae (Finke,[48] 2002)	579 g/kg	2423	5058	NA	177	43.12[52,a]	197	6.9[52]
Superworm, adult beetle (Oonincx & Dierenfeld,[58] 2012)	61.8%	NA	NA	14.25	NA	68.05	NA	NA
Waxworm (Finke,[48] 2002)	314 g/kg	2747	6619	51.4[52,a]	249	41.3[52,a]	141	6.6[52]
Silkworm (Finke,[48] 2002)	1045 g/kg	674	3896	NA	14	NA	93	NA
Earthworm (Barker,[52] 1998) Wild-caught	74.5%	NA	NA	12.6	NA	32.5[52,a]	NA	5.2[52]
Earthworm (Finke,[48] 2002) Commercial	204 g/kg or 75.8%[52]	708	4317	NA	16	50.6[52,a]	105	8.1[52]
Butterworm (Finke, 2013)	602 g/kg	2977	7479	NA	294	NA	155	NA
Black soldier fly larvae (Finke, 2012)	612 g/kg	1994	5139	NA	140	NA	175	NA
Fruit fly (Oonincx & Dierenfeld,[58] 2012)	69%	NA	NA	19	NA	68	NA	NA
Adult house fly (Finke 2012)	748	918	3643	NA	19	NA	197	NA
Turkestan roaches–nymphs (Finke,[47] 2013)	691	1602	4205	NA	100	NA	190[F13]	NA

Hissing cockroaches (Oonincx & Dierenfeld,[58] 2012)	62%	NA	24.6	NA	62.5	NA	NA
Six spotted cockroaches (Oonincx & Dierenfeld,[58] 2012)	56.6%	NA	31.2	NA	60.5	NA	NA
German cockroach (Pennino et al,[62] 1991) Wild-caught	71.2%	NA	20	NA	78.75a	NA	12.6
Wood louse (Oonincx & Dierenfeld,[58] 2012)	68%	NA	11.5	NA	41.2	NA	NA
False katydids (Oonincx & Dierenfeld,[58] 2012)	64%	NA	9	NA	77.8	NA	NA
Migratory locust (Oonincx & van der Poel,[61] 2011)	69%	21.3 kJ/g DM	NA	186	NA	649	NA
Termites (Pennino et al,[62] 1991)	78.7%	NA	6.5	NA	59.28	NA	NA
Honey bee (female/male) (Pennino et al,[62] 1991)	65.7%/72.4%	NA	10.6/10.5	NA	60/64.4a	NA	9.6/10.3
Slug (Pennino et al,[62] 1991)	85%	NA	10.7	NA	56.9a	NA	9.1
Gypsy moth (Pennino et al,[62] 1991)	68.6%	NA	44.6	NA	80a	NA	12.8
Dragonfly nymph (Pennino et al,[62] 1991)	77.9%	NA	58.5	NA	76.25a	NA	12.2
Dung beetle (Pennino et al,[62] 1991)	58.3%	NA	20.6	NA	48.75a	NA	7.8
Aquatic Invertebrates							
Krill (Pennino et al,[62] 1991)	84%	NA	3	NA	78.75a	NA	12.6
Squid (Pennino et al,[62] 1991)	80.6%	NA	10.7	NA	56.9a	NA	9.1
Crayfish (without exoskeleton) (Pennino et al,[62] 1991)	80.2%	NA	10.3	NA	66.88a	NA	10.7

a Protein calculated from available nitrogen (%DM) and multiplied by 6.25.

Data from Barker D, Fitzpatrick MP, Dierenfeld ES. Nutrient composition of selected whole invertebrates. Zoo Biol 1998;17:123–34.

Table 2
Summary of macronutrient and vitamin composition in select insect feeders

	Ca (%DM or mg/kg)	Phosphorus (%DM or mg/kg)	Vitamin A (IU/kg)[a]	Vitamin E (IU/kg)[b]	Vitamin D₃ (IU/kg)	Retinol (µg/kg DM)[a]	α-Tocopherol (µg/kg DM)[b]
House cricket (Finke,[48] 2002)	407 mg/kg	2950	<1000	19.7	<256	NA	NA
Mealworm larvae (Finke,[48] 2002)	169 mg/kg	2850	<1000	<5	<256	NA	NA
Mealworm, adult beetle (Finke,[48] 2002)	231 mg/kg	2770	<1000	<5	<256	NA	NA
Mealworm, adult beetle (Oonincx & Dierenfeld,[58] 2012)	0.06%	0.79%	12	9	NA	3.6	6
Superworm larvae (Finke,[48] 2002)	177 mg/kg	2370	<1000	7.7	<256	NA	NA
Superworm, adult beetle (Oonincx & Dierenfeld,[58] 2012)	0.06%	0.71%	41	17.8	NA	12	12
Waxworm (Finke,[48] 2002)	243 mg/kg	1950 mg/kg	<1000	13.3	<256	NA	NA
Silkworm (Finke,[48] 2002)	177 mg/kg	407 mg/kg	1580	8.9	<256	NA	NA
Earthworm (Barker et al,[52] 1998) Wild-caught	0.97%	0.79%	2400	70	NA	NA	NA
Earthworm (Finke,[48] 2002) Commercial	444 mg/kg	1590 mg/kg	<1000	NA	<256	NA	NA
Butterworm (Finke, 2012)	125 mg/kg	2250 mg/kg	NA	NA	159	<300	13
Black soldier fly larvae (Finke, 2012)	9340 mg/kg	3560 mg/kg	NA	NA	100	<300	6.2
Fruit fly (Oonincx & Dierenfeld,[58] 2012)	0.24%	1.22%	2.2	166	NA	0.7	112
Adult house fly (Finke, 2012)	765 mg/kg	3720 mg/kg	NA	NA	<20	<300	29.7
Turkestan roaches (Oonincx & Dierenfeld,[58] 2012)	0.19%	0.95%	83	17	NA	24.8	11.4

Hissing cockroaches (Oonincx & Dierenfeld,[58] 2012)	0.17%	0.57%	386	21	NA	115.8	14.2
Six spotted cockroaches (Oonincx & Dierenfeld,[58] 2012)	0.1%	0.55%	211	20	NA	63	13
German cockroach (Pennino et al,[62] 1991) Wild-caught	NA	NA	NA	NA	NA	0.3	179.3
Wood louse (Oonincx & Dierenfeld,[58] 2012)	14.38%	1.22%	NA	NA	NA	NA	NA
Migratory locust, diet of ryegrass only (Oonincx & van der Poel,[61] 2011)	0.77%–0.84%	6.52%–7.02%	NA	NA	NA	0.11 mg/kg	NA
False katydids (Oonincx & Dierenfeld,[58] 2012)	0.24%	0.90%	2953	164	NA	886 mg/kg	110 mg/kg
Termites (Pennino et al,[62] 1991)	NA	NA	NA	NA	NA	1.2	152.60
Honey bee (male/female) (Pennino et al,[62] 1991)	NA	NA	NA	NA	NA	0.93/0.85	10.4/27.1
Slug (Pennino et al,[62] 1991)	NA	NA	NA	NA	NA	1.1	15.4
Gypsy moth (Pennino et al,[62] 1991)	NA	NA	NA	NA	NA	0.1	149.3
Dragonfly nymph (Pennino et al,[62] 1991)	NA	NA	NA	NA	NA	NA	48.5
Dung beetle (Pennino et al,[62] 1991)	NA	NA	NA	NA	NA	0	154.6
Aquatic Invertebrates							
Krill (Pennino et al,[62] 1991)	NA	NA	NA	NA	NA	23.3	115.1
Squid (Pennino et al,[62] 1991)	NA	NA	NA	NA	NA	6.7	222.1
Crayfish (without exoskeleton) (Pennino et al,[62] 1991)	NA	NA	NA	NA	NA	0.2	116.2

[a] Vitamin A activity = 0.3 μg retinol = 1 IU (Olson, 1984) and 0.7 mg/kg vitamin A = 2300 IU/g vitamin A.
[b] 0.1 mg α-tocopherol = 1.49 IU vitamin E activity (Pennino, 1991).

- Krill, *Euphasia pacifica*[62]
- Squid, *Loligo pealei*[62]
- Crayfish, *Procambarus blandingi*[62]

MAJOR COMPONENTS OF NUTRITION

The National Research Council (NRC; www.nap.edu) provides an open resource for the nutrient requirements for most production and laboratory animals based on extensive review of experimental data. A database of experimentally derived nutrient requirement for herptile species does not exist. In the herptile literature, the nutrient profile of invertebrates is often compared with the minimal nutrient requirements of laboratory rats for conventional reference. Some of the nutrient components reviewed in this article will reference NRC rat minimums to highlight deficient and excessive nutritive values of select invertebrate prey.

Metabolizable Energy

Metabolizable energy (ME) is defined as the amount of net energy gained after the energy for digestion and absorption has been accounted for after a meal. This amount is largely influenced by species, age, activity, and, in a herptile's case, environmental temperature. The joules of energy required to increase basal body temperature define the maintenance requirements in rodent models. Poikilotherms do not use energy to maintain their body temperatures as mammals; therefore, herptiles require fewer calories than mammals require for maintenance.[63]

Herptile metabolic rates relate to metabolic body size. Pough and colleagues[64] offer a concise explanation for the digestive efficiency of herptiles: *"Digestive efficiency is function of diet, not of phylogentic lineage, and amphibians and reptiles extract energy and nutrients with the same efficiency as birds and mammals.[65] What does differ between endotherms and ectotherms is the rate of food processing, whereby mammals process food 10 times faster due to a comparatively enlarged gut surface area. This difference is not a handicap for herptiles, because their energy needs are about 10 times lower than those of endotherms."*

ME is measured as kilocalories per kilogram or kcal/kg. Using proximate analysis results, ME can be calculated as [(4 × gram of crude protein) + (9 × gram of crude fat) + (4 × gram of nitrogen-free extract)]. The minimum energy requirements for maintenance in mammals can be achieved in a diet of 3800 to 4100 kcal/kg. The range can vary from 112 to 311 kcal ME/body weight$_{kg}^{0.75}$ per day depending on the metabolic demands of rats, reflected during growth, lactation, or illness.

Reported values for ME in feeder insects can vary based on measurement. In older reports, ME was calculated based on a dry matter (DM) basis alone. This measurement does not account for the wide variability in energy density for the food item. DM basis, energy density defined as (DM-ED), is the most accurate and widely used method of expressing food's nutrient content [NRC 1995].[66] The DM-ED value is the ME kcal/kg divided by the % DM.

The unadjusted ME kcal/kg range for silkworms, earthworms, house crickets, and flies varies from 700 to 2700 kcal/kg, which all decrease to less than the minimal maintenance energy needs for laboratory rats if it were fed as a complete diet (see **Table 1**).[48] Martin and colleagues[41] reported mealworm ME ranges from 5600 to 5700 ME kcal/kg, which significantly exceed minimums. Mealworms fed as a sole diet item could lead to excessive growth and obesity. The energy-density–adjusted ME for black soldier fly larvae, Turkistan roaches, and butterworms range from 5139 to 7479 kcal ME/kg.[47] These values are also nearly twice the rat ME minimum for growth. **Table 1** provides energy density-adjusted ME kcal/kg values to demonstrate the importance of taking the insect's high-energy density into account when estimating ME. Most larval insects contain high-energy content that may exceed minimal requirements if fed as an exclusive diet.

Protein

The protein content of a diet reflects its amino acid composition. Protein requirements are established based on the energy concentration in the diet, amino acid composition of the protein, and bioavailability of the amino acids [NRC 1995]. The recovery of nitrogen also reflects amino acid content.[47] Most amino acids requirements can be met in highly digestible diets that contain 12% protein and 5% fat. A minimum of 7% of protein is required as fed in a natural-ingredient diet. In a 3800 to 4100 kcal ME/kg diet, this equates to a minimum of 150 g/kg protein with 10% moisture content "as fed" growth.

Few studies provide the complete amino acid profile for selected feeder insects.[40,46–48,53] Crude protein (% DM) and estimates calculated based on nitrogen recovery are more commonly reported.[47] The amino acid content of the insect's exoskeleton or cuticle has been evaluated to analyze how amino acids in the cuticle contribute to the total protein estimate.[53] The content of the cuticle is measured by acid detergent fraction (ADF) and nitrogen detergent fractions to estimate fiber and nitrogen recovery, respectively. In one study, an average of 16.6% of the ADF by weight was composed of amino acids in crickets, mealworms, silkworms, waxworms, and bee brood.[53] Given the small portion of amino acids found within the ADF, a more accurate estimate of total protein is achieved by multiplying the nitrogen recovery by 6.25.

In studies that have evaluated the total amino acid composition,[46,47,60] the sulfur group amino acids, specifically methionine and cystine, appear to be the most limiting. The NRC minimum for growth in rats for methionine is 9.8 g/kg diet and several insects fit a profile that supports meeting the minimum, on an energy basis, with the butterworm meeting 91% of the NRC recommendation.[47]

Katydids, adult crickets, houseflies, adult fruit flies, adult Hissing cockroaches, and Turkestan roaches have a relatively high protein content. The juvenile roaches have less protein and fat content than the adults.[67] The protein content is higher in the adult beetles (superworm and mealworm) than that for the larval stages.[67] The same is true for nymph crickets in comparison to adult crickets.[48] The reported total crude protein values for most of the insect feeders meet the NRC minimum requirement for rats or exceed them by 2 to 4 times (see **Table 1**). It is important to note that while the total protein estimates seem in excess of nutrient minimums, information regarding cuticle digestion and insect protein bioavailability in herptile species is limited.[1,63,68]

Fat

The lipid component of a diet provides a concentrated energy source, aids in fat-soluble vitamin absorption, provides essential fatty acids, and usually increases diet accessibility or palatability [NRC 1995]. In laboratory rats, 5% dietary lipid appears to be the optimal lipid requirement for growing rats and assures adequate vitamin A absorption. In a diet that contains 10% moisture as fed, at 3800 to 4100 kcal ME/kg, this would equate to 50 g/kg of diet fed.

Essential fatty acids, such as lineolic acid (n-6) and α-linolenic acid (n-3), are essential for growth, reproductive success, capillary membrane stability, dermatologic health, and neuronal health. For rats, maintenance recommendations for linoleic acid and α-linolenic acid are 0.5% to 1.3% (6 g/kg diet) and 0.4% (2 g/kg diet) of the dietary

ME, respectively. There are few studies that evaluate the fatty acid composition of invertebrate feeders and, among those reported, most insects contain significant quantities of oleic, linoleic, and palmitic acid.[40,46–48,60] The black soldier fly larva contains high levels of lauric acid.

Crude fat percentages reported in the commercial invertebrate prey analysis reflect values 3 to 10 times the optimal lipid requirement for rats (see **Table 1**). The larval and nymph forms of beetles and roaches contain more fat than their adult counterparts. As a rule, the roaches have a moderate to high fat content. Larval moths, adult moths, and larval beetle species have some of the highest fat contents reported, such as the waxworm (249 g/kg) and butterworm (294 g/kg). Adult houseflies, black soldier fly larva, migratory locusts, slugs, and honey bees appear to have moderate amounts of crude fat. Earthworms, silkworms, false katydids, adult fruit flies, wood louse, termites, and krill appear to have lower fat contents.

Vitamins and Mineral Content

Vitamin A
Active forms of vitamin A include retinol, retinal, 3-hydroxyretinal, and retinyl esters, whereas β-carotene is a provitamin that is usually converted into an active retinol. The absorption of vitamin A, as a fat-soluble vitamin, corresponds with an adequate lipid content in the insect's diet. Hypovitaminosis A is a common clinical problem in amphibians. Deficiencies can result in vision loss, epithelial hyperplasia, squamous metaplasia and keratinization of mucosal epithelium, growth failure, dermal ulcerations, and bone defects. In captive anurans, an inability to use the tongue effectively for prey apprehension, called "short tongue syndrome," is recognized secondary to hypovitaminosis A.[69–71] The compromise of epithelial health affords infectious diseases a window of opportunity to breech the body's largest organ and most important physical barrier used by the immune system, the integument.

The NRC minimum requirement for retinol in rats is 2300 IU/kg. In the literature, some reports of insect vitamin A levels are based on recovery of β-carotene and not specifically retinol or retinal, which are the bioavailable forms for the herptile consumer.[72] Some insects can convert ingested β-carotene into retinol, retinal, and 3-hydroxyretinal.[73] Retinal is naturally produced in the compound eye of insects. Herbivorous feeder insects, such as the false katydid, migratory locust, and silkworm, have higher retinol levels than other feeder insects. Most invertebrate species contain less than 300 µg/kg or 1000 IU/kg of retinol; however, false katydids, wild-caught earthworms, and silkworms have the reported highest contents at 2953, 2400, and 1580 IU/kg, respectively. Wild-caught termites have been reported to contain 7420 µg/kg retinol DM (see **Table 2**).[60]

Vitamin E
Often defined solely as the body's antioxidant vitamin, vitamin E requirements are commonly measured as α-tocopherol, whereby 42 µmol/kg is essential in diets containing less than 10% fat, accounting for a vitamin E content of 27 IU/kg diet or 18 mg/kg. Many invertebrate feeders meet this requirement, including the adult housefly (29.7 mg/kg),[48] adult crickets (19.7 mg/kg),[48] waxworms (13.3 mg/kg),[48] and butterworms (13.0 mg/kg).[47] However, vitamin E availability is a function of the amount and type of dietary fat. Reports of hypovitaminosis E in captive insectivores are rare; however, Dierenfeld[74] has reported vitamin E deficiencies in zoo animals that were maintained on a 50-mg to 200-mg α-tocopherol/kg diet, which significantly exceeds the 18-mg α-tocopherol/kg diet suggested by the NRC minimums for growth in rats.

Vitamin D₃

Endocrine regulation of calcium in herptile species shares similarities to mammalian species; however, the nutrient sensitivity profiles differ based on the mode of vitamin D_3 acquisition. Although ergocholecalciferol (vitamin D_2) can be ingested and used to create cholecalciferol (vitamin D_3) in some mammals, many reptiles and amphibians cannot use vitamin D_2 as a precursor for vitamin D_3. The photobiosynthesis of provitamin D_3 (7-dehydrocholesterol) to previtamin D_3 *requires* ultraviolet B (UVB) supplementation in diurnal reptiles.[75] The green iguana has historically been recognized as the best example of metabolic bone disorders secondary to the absence of UVB supplementation; however, the clinical evidence of insectivorous reptiles and amphibians exists as well.

When evaluating the minimal vitamin D_3 requirements for mammals, a 25 μg/kg or 1000 IU/kg diet is required to prevent serious disruptions in calcium homeostasis. Severe ionized calcium deficiencies can lead to several disorders, including growth retardation, pathologic fractures, hypocalcemia, osteopenia, tetany, postovulatory stasis, and seizure activity. In many of the invertebrate prey offered to captive herptile species, levels less than 256 IU/kg have been detected. One study has noted cholecalciferol levels ranging from 3 to 7 nmol/L in the Goliath bird-eating spider, *Theraphosa blondi*.[76] The cholecalciferol levels may have resulted from ingesting feeder crickets that were maintained on a supplemented diet. To date, there are no formal studies that rigorously evaluate vitamin D_3 supplementation in common feeder insects. Vitamin D_3 content was evaluated in a chicken starter diet as a gut-loading diet base for mealworms. The diet contained 675 IU vitamin D_3 and the mealworms contained 132 IU after diet exposure.[55]

Calcium and phosphorus

Calcium absorption relies on several factors, including UVB supplementation, dietary vitamin D_3, and oral calcium availability, and depends on the health status of the gastrointestinal tract, kidneys, integument, and musculoskeletal system. The body's largest reserve, the skeleton, is largely affected if nutritional deficiencies exist. Some amphibians (eg, ranid and hylid frogs) store calcium reserves in paravertebral lime sacs.[77]

The minimum requirements for several species of herptile species have been extrapolated based on the clinical onset of diseases associated with hypocalcemia. In rats, 5 g/kg calcium is required for maintenance. It is well known that most invertebrate species do not have calcium contents that come close to this requirement. There are 2 insects that are exceptions to this rule. The black soldier fly larva[47] naturally contains 9.3 g/kg without dietary supplementation and the wood louse, *P scaber*,[58] contains 14% calcium on a DM basis, accounting for a 11.79 calcium to phosphorus (Ca:P) ratio. For other invertebrates, dietary calcium supplementation before consumption is a necessity to augment their nutritive quality. Phosphorus requirements are easily met in most diets for rats, with the NRC minimal requirement at 3 g/kg diet. In most invertebrates, this minimal requirement is met or exceeded, ranging from 1.5 to 3.7 g/kg, usually demonstrating an inverse Ca:P ratio in the prey item.

CHALLENGES WITH DIGESTIBILITY AND BIOAVAILABILITY

The digestibility of an insect largely dictates the bioavailability of any nutrient. The presence of the invertebrate cuticle limits insect digestion and nutrient bioavailability in 2 major ways. First, the cuticle can serve as a digestive barrier to absorption of the gut contents of the insect. Second, the protein content of the cuticle itself may be inaccessible in herptiles that do not possess gastric enzymes and chitinases necessary to degrade the exoskeleton.

Chitinolytic digestion has been demonstrated in a limited number of amphibians.[21,78] Invertebrates have sclerotic exoskeletons composed of chitin and amino acids. Although some herptiles may have unique digestive enzymes to aid in chitin digestion, the enzyme profile may alter or prohibit the nutrient bioavailability. Allen and colleagues[2] evaluated the calcium reserves and total calcium content of wild-caught fox geckos, *Hemidactylus garnoti*, and wild-caught Cuban tree frogs, *Osteopilus septentrionalis*, that were fed calcium-supplemented crickets. Geckos fed crickets on a high-calcium cricket diet (4.02% DM cricket calcium content) maintained higher calcium composition than geckos fed a low-calcium cricket diet (3.43% DM cricket calcium content). There was no radiographic effect, measured by changes in endolymphatic calcium reserves and paravertebral lime sacs, of calcium treatment in the geckos and tree frogs. Total calcium composition decreased over time for both groups, which may have resulted from egg production in females and the absence of UVB lighting for both males and females.

Dierenfeld and King[1] demonstrated this important finding in a study that evaluated the digestibility of phoenix worms fed to Mountain chicken frogs, *L fallax*. Although phoenix worms have a naturally high Ca:P ratio, bioavailability was limited if the larva was not macerated (manually or via mastication) before ingestion. When the larva was swallowed whole, the prey passed undigested through the intestinal tract. The digestibility of the wood louse, *P scaber*, requires additional study; however, Oonincx and Dierenfeld[58] noted that the insect's exoskeleton contained 24% calcium and preliminary studies of digestibility in bearded dragons revealed that there were no exoskeleton parts found in the feces of these animals.

OPTIMIZING INSECT NUTRITIVE VALUE

Literature on insect diet manipulation became available soon after initial composition studies were published. Most composition studies revealed 2 common findings for the insects evaluated. First, most larval insects have a relatively high fat content and poor macronutrient profile. Second, most insects have an inverse Ca:P and serve as a poor dietary source of vitamin A and vitamin D_3.

There are 2 major ways the nutritive profile of select feeder insects can be improved, which include dusting or gut-loading. "Dusting" refers to coating an insect with a powdered mineral and vitamin supplement before it is fed to an insectivore. Several studies have confirmed that the dusting method is an unreliable method to maximize calcium and mineral intake because mineral attachment can vary based on insect grooming behavior.[79–82] It may also decrease prey consumption because of changes in palatability. Bilby and Widdowson[83] first recognized the correlation of calcium content in earthworms and the calcium composition in blackbirds and thrushes that consumed said earthworms attained from nearby chalky soil. The term "gut-loading" describes the method of providing feeder insects with a nutrient dense diet before presenting it for consumption. Several studies have demonstrated that the calcium content of the insect's gut could be measurably altered by its diet.[2,49–51,55–57,59,61,82–87] Today, the term gut-loading has come to mean improving the overall vitamin and mineral nutritive profile of insect prey.[43,82,84,85,88]

Calcium Supplementation

The study of dietary calcium manipulation has been reported in mealworms, crickets, silkworms, waxworms, and superworms. Mealworms have been extensively studied and the following conclusions can be made regarding gut-loading the species to reverse their poor Ca:P ratio.

Mealworms appear to avoid dietary consumption of calcium at 12% or greater in gut-loading diets; there several studies that outline calcium content improvement, but none that achieve a Ca:P of 1.66, which is the minimum nutrient requirement for rats. Guidelines for achieving the nutrient minimum can be achieved by adding 90 g/kg calcium to the base diet for 48-hour exposure before feeding the supplemented larva to the insectivores.[82] In adult crickets, 51 g/kg calcium can be added to the base diet for 48-hour exposure, and for silkworms, 23 g/kg calcium can be added to the diet can match nutrient minimums. Superworms and waxworms studies have not provided guidelines to meet nutrient minimums. In superworms, a base diet of 9% DM calcium achieves a Ca:P of 1.4 in 48 hours.[88] In waxworms, a 7.9%DM calcium diet achieved a Ca:P =1.33 in 72 hours.[59]

Vitamin A Supplementation

Insect diet manipulation studies aimed at augmenting insect vitamin A levels are scarce[58,80,82,89,90]; however, one study has validated a regression equation used to provide retinol supplementation guidelines for crickets, silkworms, and mealworms.[82] Oonincx and Dierenfeld[58] have evaluated how wheat bran and carrot supplementation may alter available β-carotene and retinol in the migratory locust. The addition of carrots increased β-carotene levels and subsequent retinol levels in both the penultimate and the adult locusts from 0.11 mg/kg DM in both groups to 0.19 mg/kg DM and 0.15 mg/kg DM retinol, respectively.

Ogilvy and colleagues[89] evaluated the carotenoid accumulation in the 3 species of crickets, *Gryllus bimaculatus*, *Gryllodes sigillatus*, and *A domesticus*, by testing a wheat-bran, fish-food–based formulated diet, and fresh fruit and vegetable diet. Cartenoid accumulation was poor in all 3 species; however, the fruit and vegetable diet provided the highest levels of retinol in the domestic cricket.[89] Attard[84] formulated a specialized cricket diet that achieves good palatability for the insect and augments all macronutrients, vitamins, and minerals to supply NRC nutrient minimums to the insectivore consumer.

In addition to the aforementioned studies, there are some clinical investigations that have reported guidelines for supplementation of vitamin A in herptile species. Dietary supplementation of vitamin A has been reported by administering 0.1 mg liver from frozen food rodents (20 μg liver = 66 IU vitamin A orally once a week) and has been used to treat periorbital squamous metaplasia secondary to hypovitaminosis A in a tiger salamander, *A tigrinum*.[71] Topical absorption studies have been performed in yellow and blue poison arrow frog, *D tinctorius*,[91] New Guinea tree frog, *Litoria infrafrenata*,[91] African foam nesting frog, *Chiromantis xerampelina*,[91,92] Puerto Rican crested toad, *Peltophryne lemur*.[91] Collective results suggest that topical application of Aquasol at 50 to 100 USP for frogs less than 20 g and 100 to 150 USP dose for frogs greater than 20 g resulted in not only the resolution of short tongue syndrome and dermal ulcerations but also significant increases in serum levels were demonstrated in the New Guinea tree frog.[91]

McComb[90] evaluated oral administration (25 IU/g body retinyl palmitate), gut-loaded crickets (70: retinyl acetate/30: retinyl palmitate mixed in water and misted on cricket food), and dusted cricket vitamin A formations (Reptivite D$_3$) in Puerto Rican crested toads, *P lemur*. After 69 days of vitamin A diet depletion and a subsequent 102 days of treatment, circulating retinol revealed that the dusting method of vitamin A supplementation may result in higher circulating retinol levels than gut-loading and oral supplementation. The same study revealed that adult cane toads, *Bufo marinus*, and Cuban tree frogs, *O septentrionalis*, could not convert dietary β-carotene to retinol, while noting that although Leopard frogs, *Rana pipiens*, can store β-carotene in the liver, little is known if or how it is used. Wright[93] has reported a vitamin A responsive reduction in the periocular swelling of Chiricahua leopard frogs, *Rana chiricahuensis*, with the use of a β-carotene-based vitamin A supplement. Parental supplementation must be provided with care, because iatrogenic hypervitaminosis[68] can occur and there are no well-documented cases in the literature.[69]

Vitamin D₃ Supplementation

The variability of a herptile's dietary and/or photobiosynthetic vitamin D_3 dependence is clinically appreciated but limited studies are available that detail the specific needs of most captive species.[2] This disparity limits the practitioner to assumptions about vitamin requirements and forces one to extrapolate based on the natural history of the species. Overall, most reptile and amphibian veterinarians recommend providing UVB exposure that is comparable to levels experienced in the animal's natural environment. This UVB exposure is commonly recommended over complete reliance on dietary supplementation for 2 reasons. First, dusting insects with a powder containing vitamin D_3 often results in an immeasurable way to account for ingestion.[94] Many insects, especially crickets, groom powders from their bodies within minutes of exposure.[55,77] Second, the amount of vitamin D_3 in marketed reptile products can be widely variable and accidental toxicity can occur.

SUMMARY

The study of amphibian nutrition still requires detailed review of species-specific natural prey analysis. Invertebrate nutrient composition has been formally studied for more than 60 years and presents the following conclusions: (1) in general, insects are poor in overall calcium content; (2) larval insects have high fat and protein component; and (3) altering the gut contents of some insects can improve their overall nutritive quality. The fat-soluble vitamin profile for most inverts is lacking. The false katydid and silkworm contain high levels of retinol. Most invertebrates have a large inverse Ca:P ratio, except for the black soldier larva and wood louse. For black soldier larva, calcium bioavailability may only be achieved by macerating the larva before ingestion in some herptile species. The bioavailability of all nutrients is highly dependent on the insectivore's ability to digest the prey's gut contents item, which can be prevented by the presence of the insect's exoskeletons. There are new guidelines for calcium and vitamin A supplementation that can help augment invertebrate nutrient profiles to match the minimum NRC requirements established for rats.

REFERENCES

1. Dierenfeld ES, King JD. Digestibility and mineral availability of phoenix worms, hermetia illucens, ingested by mountain chicken frogs, leptodactylus fallax. J Herp Med Surg 2008;18:100–5.
2. Allen ME, Oftedal OT, Ullrey DE. Effect of dietary calcium concentration on mineral composition of fox geckos (Hemidactylus garnoti) and cuban tree frogs (Osteopilus septentrionalis). J Zoo Wildl Med 1993;24:118–28.
3. Wright K. Taxonomy of amphibians kept in captivity. In: Amphibian Medicine and Captive Husbandry. Malabar (FL): Krieger Publishing; 2001. p. 3–14.
4. Sokol OM. The phylogeny of anuran larvae: a new look. Copeia 1975;1975:1–23.
5. Orton GL. The systematics of vertebrate larvae. Syst Biol 1953;2:63–75.
6. Goodman G. Oral biology and conditions of amphibians. Vet Clin North Am Exot Anim Pract 2003;6:467–75.

7. Haas A. Mandibular arch musculature of anuran tadpoles, with comments on homologies of amphibian jaw muscles. J Morphol 2001;247:1–33.

8. Duellman WE. Food and feeding. In: Duellman WE, editor. Biology of amphibians. Baltimore (MD): JHU Press; 1994. p. 229–40.

9. Reeder WG. The digestive system. In: Moore JA, editor. Physiology of the amphibia. New York: Academic Press; 1964. p. 99–149.

10. Clayton LA. Amphibian gastroenterology. Vet Clin North Am Exot Anim Pract 2005;8:227–45.

11. Zug GR, Vitt LJ, Caldwell JP. Amphibians. Herpetology: an introductory biology of amphibians and reptiles. San Diego (CA): Academic Press; 1993. p. 3–41.

12. Olsen I. Digestion and nutrition. In: Kluge AG, editor. Chordate structure and function. 2nd edition. New York: Macmillan; 1977. p. 270–305.

13. Hourdry J, Chabot JG, Menard D, et al. Intestinal brush border enzyme activities in developing amphibian Rana catesbeiana. Comp Biochem Physiol Physiol 1979;63:121–5.

14. Fanning J, Tyler M, Shearman D. Rbeobatrachus silus. Gastroenterology 1982; 82:62–70.

15. Janes RG. Studies on amphibian digestive system, IV. The effect of diet on the small intestine of rana sylvatica. Copeia 1939;1939:134–40.

16. Janes RG. Studies on the amphibian digestive system. III. The origin and development of pancreatic islands in certain species of anura. J Morphol 1938;62:375–91.

17. Janes RG. Studies on the amphibian digestive system. I. Histological changes in the alimentary tract of anuran larvae during involution. J Exp Zool 1934;67: 73–91.

18. Janes RG. Studies on the amphibian digestive system II. Comparative histology of the pancreas, following early larval development, in certain species of anura. J Morphol 1937;61:581–611.

19. Naya DE, Farfán G, Sabat P, et al. Digestive morphology and enzyme activity in the Andean toad Bufo spinulosus: hard-wired or flexible physiology? Comp Biochem Physiol A Mol Integr Physiol 2005;140:165–70.

20. Ardavin C, Zapata A, Villena A, et al. Gut-associated lymphoid tissue (GALT) in the amphibian urodele Pleurodeles waltl. J Morphol 1982;173:35–41.

21. Oshima H, Miyazaki R, Ohe Y, et al. Isolation and sequence of a novel amphibian pancreatic chitinase. Comp Biochem Physiol Biochem Mol Biol 2002;132:381–8.

22. Wright KM, Whitaker BR. Amphibian medicine and captive husbandry. Malabar (FL): Krieger Publishing Company; 2001.

23. Bragg AN. Gnomes of the night. The spadefoot toads. Philadelphia: University of Pennsylvania Press; 1965.

24. Bragg AN. Further study of predation and cannibalism in spadefoot tadpoles. Herpetologica 1964;20(1):17–24.

25. Orton GL. Dimorphism in larval mouthparts in spadefoot toads of the scaphiopus hammondi group. Copeia 1954;1954(2):97–100.

26. Altig R, Whiles MR, Taylor CL. What do tadpoles really eat? Assessing the trophic status of an understudied and imperiled group of consumers in freshwater habitats. Freshwat Biol 2007;52:386–95.

27. Schiesari L, Werner EE, Kling GW. Carnivory and resource-based niche differentiation in anuran larvae: implications for food web and experimental ecology. Freshwat Biol 2009;54:572–86.

28. Dayton GH, Wapo S. Cannibalistic behavior in Scaphiopus couchii: more evidence for larval anuran oophagy. J Herpetol 2002;36:531–2.

29. Poelman EH, Dicke M. Offering offspring as food to cannibals: oviposition strategies of amazonian poison frogs (Dendrobates ventrimaculatus). Ecol Evol 2007;21:215–27.
30. Pramuk JB, Hiler B. An investigation of obligate oophagy of Dendrobates pumilio tadpoles. Herpetological Review 1999;30:219–20.
31. Liang MF, Huang CH, Kam YC. Effects of intermittent feeding on the growth of oophagous (Chirixalus eiffingeri) and herbivorous (Chirixalus idiootocus) tadpoles from Taiwan. J Zool 2002;256:207–13.
32. Vassilieva AB, Galoyan EA, Poyarkov NA Jr. Rhacophorus vampyrus (Anura: Rhacophoridae) reproductive biology: a new type of Oophagous tadpole in Asian treefrogs. J Herpetol 2013;47:607–14.
33. Rowley JJ, Tran DT, Le DT, et al. The strangest tadpole: the Oophagous, treehole dwelling tadpole of Rhacophorus vampyrus (Anura: Rhacophoridae) from Vietnam. J Nat Hist 2012;46:2969–78.
34. Gibson RC, Buley KR. Maternal care and obligatory oophagy in Leptodactylus fallax: a new reproductive mode in frogs. Copeia 2004;2004(1):128–35.
35. Pfennig DW, Reeve HK, Sherman PW. Kin recognition and cannibalism in spadefoot toad tadpoles. Anim Behav 1993;46:87–94.
36. Walls SC, Blaustein AR. Larval marbled salamanders, Ambystoma opacum, eat their kin. Anim Behav 1995;50:537–45.
37. Kupfer A, Müller H, Antoniazzi MM, et al. Parental investment by skin feeding in a caecilian amphibian. Nature 2006;440:926–9.
38. Parker H. Viviparous caecilians and amphibian phylogeny. Nature 1956;178:250–2.
39. Wake MH, Dickie R. Oviduct structure and function and reproductive modes in amphibians. J Exp Zool 1998;282:477–506.
40. Jones L, Cooper R, Harding R. Composition of mealworm Tenebrio molitor larvae. J Zoo Wildl Med 1972;3:34–41.
41. Martin R, Rivers J, Cowgill U. Culturing mealworms as food for animals in captivity. Int Zoo Yearbk 1976;16:63–70.
42. Van Den Sande P, Van Den Bergh W. Insect colonies and hydroponic culture as a source of food for zoological gardens. Int Zoo Yearbk 1976;16:57–62.
43. Etebari K. Application of multi-vitamins as supplementary nutrients on biological and economical characteristics of silkworm Bombyx mori L. J Asia Pac Entomol 2005;8:107–12.
44. Legay JM. Recent advances in silkworm nutrition. Annu Rev Entomol 1958;3:75–86.
45. Sarker AA, Haque M, Rab M, et al. Effects of feeding mulberry leaves supplemented with different nutrients to silkworms Bombyx mori. Curr Sci 1995;69:185–8.
46. St-Hilaire S, Sheppard C, Tomberlin JK, et al. Fly prepupae as a feedstuff for rainbow trout, Oncorhynchus mykiss. J World Aquaculture Soc 2007;38:59–67.
47. Finke MD. Complete nutrient content of four species of feeder insects. Zoo Biol 2013;32:27–36.
48. Finke MD. Complete nutrient composition of commercially raised invertebrates used as food for insectivores. Zoo Biol 2002;21:269–85.
49. Finke MD, Dunham SU, Kwabi CA. Evaluation of four dry commercial gut loading products for improving the calcium content of crickets, Acheta domesticus. J Herp Med Surg 2005;15:7–12.
50. Allen ME, Oftedal OT. Dietary manipulation of the calcium content of feed crickets. J Zoo Wildl Med 1989;20:26–33.

51. Anderson SJ. Increasing calcium levels in cultured insects. Zoo Biol 2000;19: 1–9.
52. Barker D, Fitzpatrick MP, Dierenfeld ES. Nutrient composition of selected whole invertebrates. Zoo Biol 1998;17:123–34.
53. Finke MD. Estimate of chitin in raw whole insects. Zoo Biol 2007;26:105–15.
54. Fraenkel G. The nutrition of the mealworm, Tenebrio molitor L. (Tenebrionidae, Coleoptera). Physiol Zool 1950;23:92–108.
55. Klasing KC, Thacker P, Lopez MA, et al. Increasing the calcium content of mealworms (Tenebrio molitor) to improve their nutritional value for bone mineralization of growing chicks. J Zoo Wildl Med 2000;31:512–7.
56. Hunt AS, Ward AM, Ferguson G. Effects of a high calcium diet on gut loading in varying ages of crickets (Acheta domestica) and mealworms (Tenebrio molitor). Proc Nutrition Advisory Group 4th Conference on Zoo and Wild Nutr. 2001. p. 94–102.
57. Zwart P, Rulkens RJ. Improving the calcium content of mealworms. Int Zoo Yearbk 1979;19:254–5.
58. Oonincx D, Dierenfeld E. An investigation into the chemical composition of alternative invertebrate prey. Zoo Biol 2012;31:40–54.
59. Strzelewicz MA, Ullrey DE, Schafer SF, et al. Feeding insectivores: increasing the calcium content of wax moth (Galleria mellonella) larvae. J Zoo Wildl Med 1985;16:25–7.
60. Oyarzun SE, Crawshaw GJ, Valdes EV. Nutrition of the Tamandua: nutrient composition of termites (Nasutitermes spp.) and stomach contents from wild Tamanduas (Tamandua tetradactyla). Zoo Biol 1996;15:509–24.
61. Oonincx DG, van der Poel AF. Effects of diet on the chemical composition of migratory locusts (Locusta migratoria). Zoo Biol 2011;30:9–16.
62. Pennino M, Dierenfeld ES, Behler JL. Retinol, α-tocopherol and proximate nutrient composition of invertebrates used as feed. Int Zoo Yearbk 1991;30: 143–9.
63. Donoghue SS. Nutrition of reptiles. In: Hand MS, editor. Small animal clinical nutrition. 5th edition. Topeka (KS): Mark Morris Institute; 2010. p. 1237–54.
64. Pough F, Andrews R, Cadle J, et al. Diets, foraging, and interactions with parasites and predators. Herpetology. 3rd edition. Upper Saddle River (NJ): Prentice-Hall; 2001. p. 530–66.
65. Karasov WH, Diamond JM. Interplay between physiology and ecology in digestion: Intestinal nutrient transporters vary within and between species according to diet. BioScience 1988;38:602–11.
66. Nutrient Requirements for the Laboratory Rat. In: The National Research Council, editor. Nutrient Requirements of Laboratory Animals. 4th revised edition. Washington, DC: The National Academy Press; 1995. p. 11–79.
67. Oonincx DG, van de Wal MD, Bosch G, et al. Blood vitamin D3 metabolite concentrations of adult female bearded dragons (Pogona vitticeps) remain stable after ceasing UVb exposure. Comp Biochem Physiol Biochem Mol Biol 2013; 165:196–200.
68. Donoghue S. Nutrition. In: Mader D, editor. Reptile medicine and surgery. 2nd edition. St Louis (MO): Elsevier; 2006. p. 251–98.
69. Pessier A. Short tongue syndrome and hypovitaminosis A. In: Mader DR, Divers SJ, editors. Current therapy in reptile medicine and surgery. St Louis (MO): Elsevier Health Sciences; 2013. p. 271–6.
70. Pessier A, Roberts D, Linn M. Short tongue syndrome, lingual squamous metaplasia and suspected hypovitaminosis A in captive Wyoming toads, Bufo baxteri.

9th Annual Meeting of the Association of Reptilian and Amphibian Veterinarians. Reno (NV): Association of Reptilian and Amphibian Veterinarians; 2002.

71. Kummrow M, Tseng F, Pessier AP. What is your diagnosis? Periocular swelling in Ambystoma tigrinum. J Herp Med Surg 2006;16:144–6.

72. Ross AC. Vitamin A: nutritional aspects of retinoids and carotenoids. In: Zempleni J, Galloway JR, McCormick DB, et al, editors. Handbook of vitamins. 4th edition. Boca Raton (FL): CRC Press; 2007. p. 1–40.

73. von Lintig J, Vogt K. Filling the gap in vitamin A research: molecular identification of an enzyme cleaving to β-carotene to retinal. J Biol Chem 2000;275: 11915–20.

74. Dierenfeld E. Vitamin E deficiency in zoo reptiles, birds and ungulates. J Zoo Wildl Med 1989;20:3–11.

75. Klaphake E. A fresh look at metabolic bone diseases in reptiles and amphibians. Vet Clin North Am Exot Anim 2010;13:375–92.

76. Zachariah TT, Mitchell MA. Vitamin D3 in the hemolymph of goliath bird eater spiders (Theraphosa blondi). J Zoo Wildl Med 2009;40:344–6.

77. Dacke C. Calcium regulation in sub-mammalian vertebrates. London: Academic Press; 1979.

78. Oshima H, Miyazaki R, Ohe Y, et al. Molecular cloning of a putative gastric chitinase in the toad Bufo japonicus. Zool Sci 2002;19:293–7.

79. Sullivan K, Livingston S, Valdes E. Vitamin A supplementation via cricket dusting: the effects of dusting fed and fasted crickets of three sizes using two different supplements on nutrient content. Proc Am Assoc Zoo Vet/Am Assoc Wildl Vet/Am Zoo Aquar Assoc Nutr Advisory Group Joint Conf. Tulsa (OK), 2009. p. 113.

80. Li H, Vaughan MJ, Browne RK. A complex enrichment diet improves growth and health in the endangered Wyoming toad (Bufo baxteri). Zoo Biol 2009;28: 197–213.

81. Trusk A, Crissey S. Comparison of calcium and phosphorus levels in crickets fed a high calcium diet versus those dusted with supplement. Proceedings of the Sixth and Seventh Dr Scholl Conferences on the Nutrition of Captive Wild Animals. Chicago: Lincoln Park Zoological Gardens; 1987. p. 93–9.

82. Finke MD. Gut loading to enhance the nutrient content of insects as food for reptiles: a mathematical approach. Zoo Biol 2003;22:147–62.

83. Bilby LW, Widdowson EM. Chemical composition of growth in nestling blackbirds and thrushes. Br J Nutr 1971;25:127–34.

84. Attard L. The development and evaluation of a gut-loading diet for feeder crickets formulated to provide a balanced nutrient source for insectivorous amphibians and reptiles. Animal and poultry science. Guelph (Ontario): University of Guelph; 2013.

85. Hunt Coslik AW, McClements RD. Gut loading as a method to effectively supplement crickets with calcium and vitamin A. Proceedings of the 8th conference on Zoo and Wildlife Nutrition, AZA Nutrition Advisory Group. Tulsa (OK), 2009. p. 163–71.

86. McClements RD, Slifka KA. Calcium and insect gut-loading: the development of a protocol for achieving the best Ca:P ratio for insectivorous animals. Proceedings of the Fifth Conference on Zoo and Wildlife Nutrition, 2003. p. 80.

87. Winn D, Dunham S, Mikulski S. Food for insects and insects as food: viable strategies for achieving adequate calcium. J Wildl Rehabil 2003;26:4–13.

88. Latney LT, Wyre N. Evaluation of the nutrient composition of Tenebrio molitor and Zophobas morio fed supplemental diets utilized to improve the nutrition of

insectivorous animals. 2009 Proceedings of the Annual Conference of the Association of Reptilian and Amphibian Veterinarians. Milwaukee (WI): Omnipress; 2009. p. 173.

89. Ogilvy V, Fidgett AL, Preziosi RF. Differences in carotenoid accumulation among three feeder-cricket species: implications for carotenoid delivery to captive insectivores. Zoo Biol 2012;31:470–8.

90. McComb A. Evaluation of Vitamin A Supplementations for Captive Amphibian Species. Animal Science/Nutrition. Raleigh (NC): North Carolina State University; 2010. p. 113.

91. Fleming GVE. Hypovitaminosis A in a captive collection of amphibians. Proceedings of the American Association of Zoo Veterinarians and Association of Reptile and Amphibian Veterinarians Joint Conference 2008. p. 6–8.

92. Sim RR, Sullivan KE, Valdes EV, et al. A comparison of oral and topical vitamin A supplementation in African foam-nesting frogs (Chiromantis xerampelina). J Zoo Wildl Med 2010;41:456–60.

93. Wright K. Advances that impact every amphibian patient. Exotic DVM 2005;7:82.

94. Donoghue S. Nutrition of pet amphibians and reptiles. Semin Avian Exot Pet 1998;7:148–53.

Update on Common Nutritional Disorders of Captive Reptiles

Christoph Mans, DVM[a],*, Jana Braun, DVM[b]

KEYWORDS

- Nutritional secondary hyperparathyroidism • Hypovitaminosis A • Obesity
- Dehydration • Constipation • Hypothyroidism

KEY POINTS

- Nutritional secondary hyperparathyroidism is the most important nutritional disorder in captive reptiles and is either caused by a deficiency in dietary calcium and/or vitamin D_3 or inadequate exposure to UV-B radiation.
- Hypovitaminosis A is predominately a disorder of omnivorous and carnivorous reptiles that receive insufficient dietary vitamin A. Herbivorous reptiles rarely suffer from this disorder because of their ability to endogenously synthetize vitamin A from plant-derived provitamins contained in their diet.
- Nutritional secondary hypothyroidism caused by excessive intake of goiterogenic plants is predominately a disorder of herbivorous reptiles. The diagnosis should be made carefully because evaluation of thyroid function has not been reported in reptiles and visualization of the thyroid gland may be challenging because of the intracoelomic location of the gland.

INTRODUCTION

Nutritional disorders of captive reptiles remain very common despite the increasing knowledge about reptile husbandry and nutrition. Many nutritional disorders are diagnosed late in the disease process and often secondary complications have occurred. Therefore, every attempt should be made to educate reptile owners and keepers about the proper care and, in particular, dietary needs of reptiles under their care because all nutritional disorders seen in captive reptiles are preventable.

However, because the class Reptilia is so diverse and reptiles have adapted to such a large variety of climates, habitats, and natural diets, making general applicable

[a] Special Species Health Service, Department of Surgical Sciences, School of Veterinary Medicine, University of Wisconsin, 2015 Linden Drive, Madison, WI 53706, USA; [b] VCA Silver Lake Animal Hospital, 10726 19th Avenue Southeast, Everett, WA 98208, USA
* Corresponding author.
E-mail address: cmans@vetmed.wisc.edu

Vet Clin Exot Anim 17 (2014) 369–395
http://dx.doi.org/10.1016/j.cvex.2014.05.002
1094-9194/14/$ – see front matter © 2014 Elsevier Inc. All rights reserved.

recommendations challenging. A detailed knowledge about the natural habitat and diet of reptiles commonly seen by veterinarians is important in order to provide the appropriate advice to reptile owners and keepers. Although the recommendations on appropriate captive diets for reptiles are based predominately on experience and anecdotal information, a growing body of scientifically derived knowledge is available to support dietary and husbandry recommendations. This article attempts to summarize the current information on the most common nutritional disorders of reptiles. Excellent reviews on basic nutrition of reptiles have been published in the literature.[1,2] The reader is encouraged to use this article as a supplement and update to the existing literature.

NUTRITIONAL SECONDARY HYPERPARATHYROIDISM

Nutritional secondary hyperparathyroidism (NSHP) in captive reptiles occurs because of dietary calcium and/or vitamin D_3 deficiencies. Deficiencies in vitamin D_3 (cholecalciferol) can occur because of insufficient dietary intake in nonherbivorous reptile species or in most cases because of a lack of adequate exposure to UV-B radiation, which is required for endogenous vitamin D_3 synthesis. NSHP is the most common nutritional disorder of captive reptiles, particularly in lizards and chelonians as well as herbivorous and insectivorous species. Animals feeding exclusively on whole prey (ie, snakes) are not affected by NSHP because whole vertebrate prey contains adequate amounts of calcium and vitamin D_3.

Bone is the major storage site of body calcium, with about 99% of body calcium stored. Vitamin D_3, calcitonin, and parathyroid hormone (PTH) control storage and release of calcium from the bone.[3] Chronic reduced blood calcium levels will trigger increased secretion of PTH from the parathyroid glands, resulting in hyperparathyroidism. Increased secretion of PTH leads to increased resorption of calcium from the bones, resulting in osteomalacia (syn fibrous osteodystrophy, nutrition-related metabolic bone disease).

Dietary factors that can lead to NSHP include insufficient calcium intake; inappropriate calcium/phosphorous (Ca:P) ratio of the diet; insufficient calcium absorption from the intestine, which is vitamin D_3 dependent; insufficient dietary vitamin D intake; or insufficient exposure to UV-B radiation (280–315 nm). The biological active form of vitamin D_3 is 1,25-dihydroxycholecalciferol (calcitriol), which regulates calcium metabolism predominately by increasing intestinal calcium absorption and renal calcium reabsorption.[3] UV-B is necessary to activate the cholecalciferol pathway in species that rely not on dietary vitamin D_3 intake, which is the case in herbivorous reptiles. If vitamin D_3 is predominately of dietary origin or endogenously synthetized differs between reptile species based on their nutritional (carnivorous, omnivorous, herbivorous) strategy and natural behavior (eg, nocturnal vs diurnal) and natural habitat.

Effect of UV-B Radiation

In omnivorous and carnivorous reptiles, the need for provision of artificial UV-B radiation in captivity remains controversial. In most reptile species evaluated, exposure to UV-B radiation will lead to increased plasma vitamin D levels. Exposure to artificial UV-B in panther chameleons (*Furcifer pardalis*) had a significant effect on plasma 25-hydroxycholecalciferol.[4] Red-eared sliders (*Trachemys scripta elegans*) had significantly higher plasma 25-hydroxycholecalciferol concentrations if turtles were exposed to artificial UV-B radiation for 4 weeks.[5] In corn snakes, exposure to artificial UV-B radiation for 4 weeks significantly increased plasma 25-hydroxycholecalciferol levels.[6] In contrast, exposing ball pythons (*Python regius*) to artificial UV-B radiation for 70 days had no significant effect on 25-hydroxycholecalciferol or ionized calcium levels.[7] As a nocturnal species, ball pythons might not need to use UV-B radiation for synthesis of cholecalciferol as compared with diurnal species.[7] In addition, dietary intake of vitamin D_3 affects basking behavior and, therefore, exposure to UV-B radiation.[4] Panther chameleons adapt their basking behavior and exposure to UV-B radiation based on their dietary vitamin D_3 intake. Chameleons with less dietary vitamin D_3 intake spend more time basking.[4]

It needs to be remembered that most forms of artificial UV-B radiation provided in captivity are only an inadequate supplement for natural sunlight that most reptiles are exposed to in their natural habitat. Hermann's tortoises (*Testudo hermanni*) exposed for 35 days to either mercury or fluorescent UV-B radiation–emitting light bulbs had significantly lower 25-hydroxycholecalciferol plasma levels compared with day 0, whereas tortoises exposed to natural sunlight maintained their plasma 25-hydroxycholecalciferol levels.[8] In bearded dragons (*Pogona vitticeps*), dietary supplementation of vitamin D_3, even at high doses, was insufficient to maintain plasma 25-hydroxycholecalciferol levels compared with bearded dragons exposed to artificial UV-B radiation.[9]

Dietary Calcium Intake

Chronic dietary calcium deficiency or excessive phosphorous intake (improper Ca:P ratio) will lead to NSHP.[10] Herbivorous reptiles with a natural diet of scrubs and grasses are frequently ingesting diets in captivity that are too high in phosphorous and low in calcium. Most commercially available insect prey species fed to reptiles have an inversed Ca:P ratio and are deficient in vitamin D_3, predisposing insectivorous reptiles to NSHP unless supplemented.[2] Therefore, supplementation in the form of gut loading and dusting is required to achieve an appropriate Ca:P ratio of at least 1:1. Pinhead-sized crickets have a balanced Ca:P ratio but are too small for many adult insectivore reptiles to be considered as a food source.[11] Although phoenix worms, which are larva of the black soldier fly (*Hermetia illucens*), also have an appropriate Ca:P ratio of 2.6:1.0, digestibility is a concern.[12] The availability and digestibility of calcium is significantly higher in phoenix worms with the exoskeleton destroyed compared with intact worms.[12] The wood lice (Porcellio scaber), a terrestrial crustacean is another invertebrate with a remarkably high Ca:P ratio, due to their mineralized exoskeleton, which contains up to 24% calcium.[13] Although the bioavailability of the calcium in wood lice is currently unknown, this species of invertebrate prey should be considered as a suitable high-calcium food source in reptiles.[13] Earthworms are another invertebrate food source, which provide a balanced Ca:P ratio (1.4:1.0). But differences between commercially available and wild earthworms have been reported. These differences are in the Ca:P ratio and also in vitamin A content and are likely related to the soil and diet earthworms ingest.[11]

Clinical signs

Clinical signs of calcium deficiency can be variable. Lethargy, reduced appetite, constipation, dystocia, or preovulatory stasis can be seen in animals with calcium deficiencies. However, these clinical signs are nonspecific, and other disease processes or husbandry problems should be ruled out. Skeletal deformities or fractures caused by demineralization of the bones are common in reptiles with calcium deficiencies (**Figs. 1** and **2**). Fractures of the limbs and ribs are most commonly seen in lizards (see **Figs. 1** and **2**). Demineralization of the mandible and maxilla will lead to deformities as well as increased flexibility (rubber jaw) (see **Fig. 1**). The shell of chelonians can be poorly mineralized and deformed.

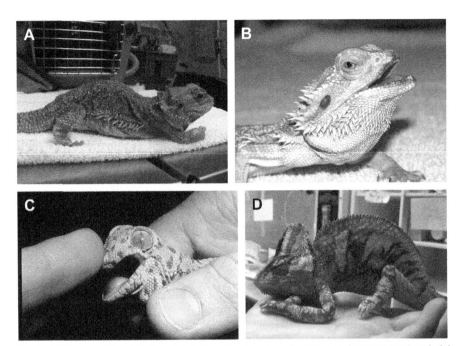

Fig. 1. NSHP in reptiles. (*A*) Skeletal deformities in a bearded dragon (*Pogona vitticeps*). (*B*) Deformation of the mandible in a bearded dragon. (*C*) Demineralization of the maxilla in a Tokay gecko (*Gecko gecko*). (*D*) Deformation and fractures of the limbs in a veiled chameleon (*Chamaeleo calyptratus*). Note the swelling of the left lower leg and the abnormal placement of the forelimbs. (*Courtesy of* [*A*] M. Pinkerton, DVM, DACVP, Madison, WI; and [*B, C*] Special Species Health Service, School of Veterinary Medicine, University of Wisconsin, Madison, WI.)

Once total body calcium stores are depleted enough, so that blood calcium levels cannot be maintained at adequate levels, muscle twitching, tremors, paresis, and neurologic signs can be seen. These clinical signs are consistent with hypocalcemic crisis, which is considered an acute decompensation of chronic NSPH.

Diagnosis
A thorough history is critical and will often allow for the identification of incorrect husbandry and dietary practices leading to NSHP and related disorders.

Plasma calcium levels are of little to no diagnostic value when assessing total body calcium and diagnosis of NSHP because of the complex homeostatic mechanisms that control blood calcium levels. Further estrogen in female reptiles can increase total blood calcium, even if an animal has NSHP. In most reptiles with NSHP, total blood calcium levels are usually still within reported reference ranges. Therefore, making conclusions and a diagnosis of calcium deficiency should be avoided without further evidence obtained, for example, by diagnostic imaging. In the case of an acute hypocalcemic crisis, total blood calcium can be diagnostic, confirming the clinical suspicion. Ionized calcium should be measured whenever possible in cases presenting with muscle tremors, depression, or seizure-like activity. For most reptile species, ionized calcium reference ranges are not available. Mean ionized calcium in green iguanas is 1.47 mmol/L ($\pm$0.105 mmol/L).[14] Assessing the total Ca:P ratio in the blood is important. A ratio of equal or smaller than 1:1 is of concern and is often associated with NSHP or renal secondary hyperparathyroidism.

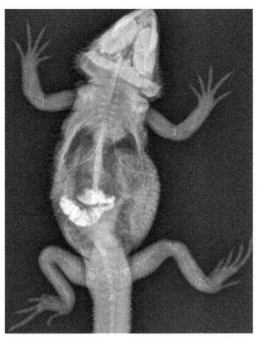

Fig. 2. NSHP in reptiles. Dorsoventral whole-body radiograph of a bearded dragon (*Pogona vitticeps*). Note the demineralization of the bones as well as fractures.

Plasma 25-hydroxycholecalciferol can be measured, and reference values for some species are available.[5,15] Levels of 25-hydroxycholecalciferol did not vary significantly between seasons in *Testudo spp*, but females had lower values than males.[15]

Radiography allows for evaluation of bone quality, degree of demineralization evaluation of fractures, and skeletal deformities. However, 40% to 50% of the bone's mineralization must be depleted before radiographic changes are detectable.[16] The use of dual-energy x-ray absorptiometry (DXA) in the green iguana showed appreciable differences in the bone density between diseased and nondiseased animals, although differences existed based on body weight.[17] DXA has also been used in Hermann's tortoises (*Testudo hermanni*) to evaluate mineral bone density.[10] DXA may be useful to monitor the response to treatment in reptiles diagnosed with reduced total body calcium stores.[3,10] DXA was also used to validate bone density of plain radiographs and correlating the measured optical densities of various skeletal structures to the density of an aluminum wedge. The optical density of the femur, measured in millimeters of aluminum equivalents, correlated highly with the total mineral bone density measured by DXA.[18]

Treatment
Parenteral administration of calcium is only indicated if a reptile presents in acute hypocalcemic crisis with clinical signs, such as muscle tremors or twitching. Calcium gluconate (50–100 mg/kg) should be administered diluted by subcutaneous, intramuscular, or intravenous administration. Repeated parenteral administration should be limited because of the risk of metastatic tissue calcification but may need to be administered repeatedly if clinical signs reoccur (eg, muscle tremors).

Once clinical improvement has occurred and patients are stable, oral calcium supplementation should be initiated. Calcium glubionate (20–50 mg/kg by mouth every 24 hours) should be administered. Alternatively, calcium carbonate can be administered if calcium glubionate is not available.

The administration of vitamin D_3 in cases of NSHP is controversial because of the risk of intoxication and metastatic calcification of tissues. In most cases of NSHP, exposure to UV-B radiation is preferred over the administration of vitamin D. In cases in which the liver or kidney function may be impaired and endogenous vitamin D_3 synthesis might be impaired, the administration of biological active vitamin D_3 (calcitriol 100–400 IU/kg intramuscularly [IM], subcutaneously [SC] or orally every 7 days for 2–3 doses) should be considered. However, because of the risks of hypervitaminosis D, the authors do not recommend to routinely administer vitamin D_3 to reptiles diagnosed with NSHP.

Identification of concurrent and secondary disorders, such as dehydration or secondary bacterial or parasitic infections, is important to aid in recovery.

Prevention

Growing reptiles and reproductive activate female reptiles have the highest calcium requirements. Offering a diet with an appropriate Ca:P ratio is critical. Calcium carbonate is the preferred form of calcium for supplementation, which can be supplemented as a powder or in the form of cuttlefish bones (**Fig. 3**). Calcium phosphate (ie, bone meal) should be avoided. Supplementation of calcium in herbivorous reptiles, such as tortoises, might not be indicated if an appropriate diet is fed.[10]

Dusting of feeder insects with calcium carbonate and/or multivitamin powders just before being offered to a predator reptile is a commonly used method to attempt to correct nutritional imbalances of most feeder insects. However, dusting can provide variable results because the amounts adhered to the insects and the change in palatability might affect the overall intake of the supplemented nutrients.[19]

Gut loading is considered a more effective method to increase the nutritional balance of feeder insects offered to insectivorous reptiles.[19] By offering a nutrient dense diets to feeder insects, the diet will be retained in the insects' gastrointestinal tract and then be ingested by reptiles. In crickets, feeding diets containing different levels of

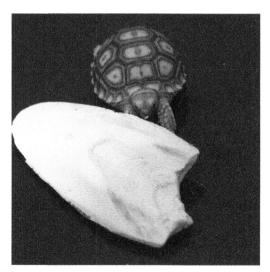

Fig. 3. Juvenile African spurred tortoise (*Centrochelys sulcata*) ingesting a cuttlefish bone during an examination at a veterinary hospital.

calcium resulted in a linear increase of calcium content in the crickets.[19] Guidelines for nutrient concentrations required for gut-loading formulas for various invertebrate diets are available.[19] Several highly palatable and nutritionally balanced invertebrate diets (eg, Orange Cube Complete Cricket Diet, Fluker Farms, Port Allen, LA) are readily available and provide a source of hydration as well as critical nutrients, leading to improved nutritional values of gut-loaded feeder insects.

Excessive supplementation with vitamin D_3 will lead to metastatic tissue calcification.[20] Juvenile leopard tortoises (*Stigmochelys pardalis*), a herbivore species, supplemented with vitamin D_3 (400 IU per kilogram of fresh weight of a vegetable mix), developed metastatic mineralization of the connective tissue of the lungs, stomach, and blood vessels, which was more pronounced in the tortoises that were supplemented with high levels of calcium carbonate.[21] Therefore, dietary vitamin D_3 supplementation, which is added in bulk to a diet and not controlled, should be avoided, particularly in herbivorous reptiles because their natural diet does not contain vitamin D_3.

Exposure to adequate amounts and wavelengths of UV-B radiation is important particularly in herbivore reptiles. Different materials commonly used in reptile enclosures can lead to the reduction of UV-B radiation (acrylic, glass, wire).[22] Therefore, it is critical that no glass or acrylic is placed between the reptile and the UV-B–emitting light source (**Fig. 4**). The output of UV-B–emitting light bulbs can be measured with a UV meter (**Fig. 5**). Exposure to direct unfiltered sunlight is preferred over artificial UV-B radiation whenever possible.

VITAMIN A–RELATED DISORDERS

Vitamin A is essential for many biological processes, such as vision, growth, reproduction, and immune function.[23] The most commonly recognized effect is its function in maintaining normal epithelial tissue. *Vitamin A* is a term used to group several preformed biological active compounds (retinol, retinal, and retinoic acid), which are only found in animal tissue, not in plants.[23,24] Precursors (provitamins) of vitamin A found in plants are termed *carotenoids*. Beta-carotene is considered the most important precursor of vitamin A.[24] However, reptiles do not seem to absorb beta-carotenes well; increased dietary beta-carotene intake has no effect on plasma beta-carotene or

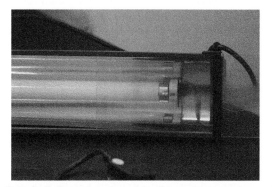

Fig. 4. Fluorescent light bulb fixture marketed for fish tanks. Note the acrylic cover, which is intended to protect the bulb from water. This fixture had been used with a UV-B–emitting fluorescent bulb in a veiled chameleon enclosure (*Chamaeleo calyptratus*). The animal was diagnosed with NSHP caused by the lack of UV-B radiation because acrylic and glass will filter out UV-B radiation.

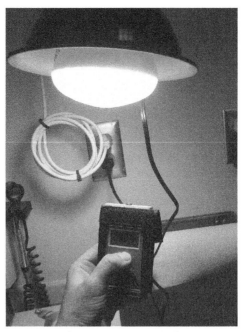

Fig. 5. Measuring UV-B output of a mercury vapor bulb using a UV meter. (*Courtesy of* J. Mayer, DVM, Athens, GA.)

vitamin A levels.[25] However, other carotenoids, such as lutein and canthaxanthin, have been recommended as more effective forms of provitamin A in reptiles.[25,26]

The amount of carotenoids present in plant material is proportional to the depth of the color of the green and yellow pigment in the plants.[24] The concentration of carotenoids in plants varies considerably with geographic location, maturity, and duration and length of storage, making it one of the most variable dietary nutrients.[23] Carotenoids are absorbed from the intestine after digestive processes make them available. Although the absorption of carotenoids is likely occurring in most animals, activation of the provitamins into vitamin A is not occurring in many carnivorous and omnivorous animals species because of the lack of the needed enzymes.[23] However, herbivorous reptiles are able to endogenously synthesize vitamin A from dietary carotenoids; therefore, a vitamin A deficiency is very uncommon in herbivorous reptiles.

The liver serves as a source of stored vitamin A and can serve as a source for at least 10 months in humans.[27,28] Therefore, it may take months before clinical signs develop secondarily in insufficient vitamin A intake.

HYPOVITAMINOSIS A

Hypovitaminosis A is a common disorder of semiaquatic turtles (eg, red-eared sliders), North American box turtles (*Terrapene* spp), and insectivorous reptiles, such as chameleons and geckos. The replacement of normal cuboidal or columnar epithelial cells (eg, in the mucosa, gland ducts) with stratified keratinizing epithelium, which is replaced in increased frequency, is the hallmark feature of hypovitaminosis A in reptiles as well as other animals. The occurring multifocal squamous metaplasia and hyperkeratosis of the epithelium of many organs will lead to clinical disease. The continued desquamation of cells leads to the accumulation of desquamated debris and predisposes to secondary infections of the periocular tissue, upper respiratory tract, and oral cavity.

Clinical Signs

Clinical signs attributed to hypovitaminosis A can be unspecific, such as reduced growth, lethargy, anorexia, and upper respiratory infections. In semiaquatic turtles, such as red-eared sliders, the most common and characteristic signs of hypovitaminosis A are blepharedema; conjunctivitis (**Fig. 6**A); and, in chronic cases, accumulation of desquamated debris within the conjunctival sacs (see **Fig. 6**B, C).[29] Often these periocular lesions are bilateral, and the resultant loss of vision will lead to anorexia. The swelling and closure of the eyelids, particularly in turtles and chameleons with vitamin A deficiency, occurs secondary to metaplasia and expansion of the anteromedial harderian gland as well as the posterolateral lacrimal gland.[1,30] Because of the swelling of the glands, the eyelids cannot be opened properly; together with increased desquamation, this will lead to the accumulation of debris in the conjunctival sac. Secondary bacterial infections are common, and it is important to identify and correct the primary underlying hypovitaminosis A in order to resolve the secondary infection.

Oral lesions, such as ulcerations and plaque formation of the tongue and buccal mucosa, as well as stomatitis and glossitis have also been linked to insufficient dietary vitamin A intake.[31,32]

In panther chameleons, clinical signs associated with a diet low in vitamin A included periocular edema, ocular discharge, swelling of the lips and gular region,

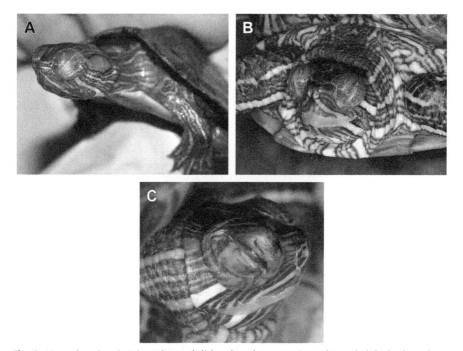

Fig. 6. Hypovitaminosis A in red-eared sliders (*Trachemys scripta elegans*). (*A*) Blepharedema and accumulation of desquamated debris in the conjunctival sac in a juvenile turtle. (*B*) Bilateral blepharedema and conjunctivitis. (*C*) Accumulation of desquamated debris in the left conjunctival sac.

tail tip necrosis, reduced reproduction, and skeletal abnormalities (ie, vertebral kinking).[33]

Although is has been proposed that the squamous metaplasia of the eustachian tubes and tympanic membrane caused by vitamin A deficiency leads to aural abscesses in turtles, there is currently no evidence to support this assumption.[34] Aural abscesses are likely multifactorial in nature, and the influence of environmental factors is yet to be fully described.

Dysecdysis and hemipenile impactions have also been associated with hypovitaminosis A but are rarely the sole clinical signs of this deficiency.

In severe cases of vitamin A deficiency, multifocal metaplasia of the epithelium and subsequent blockage with desquamated debris of the internal organs, such as the kidneys, ureters, and pancreas, can lead to systemic disease and organ failure.[1,31] In crocodiles fed a vitamin A–deficient diet, squamous metaplasia and hyperkeratosis of the renal tubules developed, leading to visceral and renal gout.[32]

Diagnosis

The dietary history and clinical sign are often sufficient to establish the diagnosis of hypovitaminosis A is reptiles. Confirming this diagnosis can be challenging; therefore, the response to treatment with beta-carotenes or vitamin A is often used to confirm the diagnosis in most captive reptiles.[29] The liver is the major storage site of vitamin A, and liver biopsies can be used to determine the hepatic vitamin A levels. Hepatic vitamin A levels for carnivorous reptiles, such as monitor lizards and snakes, have been reported to be greater than 1000 IU/g but can be much less in herbivorous reptiles, such as Testudo hermanni (10–80 IU/g).[31] Plasma retinol levels have been investigated in reptiles to diagnose vitamin A deficiency.[29] However, differences between plasma retinol levels between genders as well as differences in methodologies of measurement and reported units can make interpretation of plasma retinol levels challenging.[35] In captive aquatic turtles, the plasma retinol levels are 0.03 to 0.364 µg/mL and 0.034 to 0.415 µg/mL in tortoises (µg/0.3 = IU).[26] Plasma retinol levels in lizards and snakes have been reported between 0.049 to 0.372 µg/mL and 0.012 to 0.049 µg/mL, respectively.[26] The mean plasma retinol levels in green iguanas fed a carotenoid-deficient diet for 56 days were 0.052 ± 0.012 µg/mL.[25]

Treatment

Hypovitaminosis A is virtually impossible to develop in herbivorous reptiles unless they are anorexic for several months, which would lead to depletion of the liver vitamin A stores. Therefore, the diagnosis of hypovitaminosis A in herbivorous reptiles should be made very cautiously, and parenteral or oral administration of retinols should be avoided. Particularly in tortoises, the administration of retinols should be avoided because of the high risk of intoxication. Instead, increasing dietary carotenoids should be considered.

For omnivorous, carnivorous, and insectivorous reptiles, the dosage recommendations for vitamin A have been made largely based on extrapolation and anecdotal reports.

The following has been recommended: 500 to 5000 IU/kg IM every 7 to 14 days for up to 4 treatments.[2,29] Oversupplementation with vitamin A can occur regardless of the route of administration; therefore, oral administration does not provide a safer alternative.[36,37]

Secondary infection should be treated accordingly. Accumulated debris in the conjunctival sacs should be removed under sedation.

Prevention

Omnivorous or carnivorous reptiles should be fed whole prey (eg, mice, fish) or should be fed a commercial balanced diet (eg, aquatic turtle pellets). Feeding muscle meat or removing the internal organs of prey should be avoided because the liver is the primary storage site for retinols in the body.

Invertebrates contain only low amounts of vitamin A.[11] Therefore, they should be gut loaded. Offering diets high in carotenes will significantly increase the carotene content of the cricket.[38] However, it remains unknown whether the provided carotenes can be converted by insectivorous reptiles into biological active vitamin A.

Herbivorous reptiles being fed a plant-based diet are very unlikely to become vitamin A deficient because plants contain high amounts of carotenoids and herbivorous reptiles are able to absorb and convert carotenoids into biological active vitamin A.

HYPERVITAMINOSIS A

Intoxication with vitamin A in reptiles is always iatrogenic. Herbivorous reptiles, particularly tortoises, seem to be particularly prone to hypervitaminosis A following the administration of retinols, often given because of a suspected and, in most cases, misdiagnosed vitamin A deficiency.[31,39] However, in any reptile species hypervitaminosis A can be induced if excessive vitamin A is administered repeatedly or more than the recommended dosages.[29] The administration of a single or repeated dose of 5000 to 10,000 IU/kg parentally to aquatic turtles is safe; however, concurrent increased dietary intake, such as increased feeding of raw liver, can induce hypervitaminosis A.

Clinical Signs

Clinical signs are initially usually limited to the integument. Characteristic signs include excessive flaking of the skin, which progresses to widespread epidermal ulceration and sloughing that results in exposure of the underlying dermis (**Fig. 7**).[29] Secondary bacterial and fungal infections of the exposed dermis are common. Anorexia, lethargy and dehydration, and death are common complications.

Diagnosis

The diagnosis is based on the history of recent vitamin A administration or feeding excessive amounts of raw liver as well as the physical examination finding of widespread epidermal sloughing.

Treatment

Once vitamin A intoxication has occurred, it cannot be reversed. The focus of the therapy in such cases is on supportive care and prevention or treatment of secondary fungal and bacterial infections of the skin. Systemic and topical administration of antimicrobials is indicated. The damaged skin should be managed topically with hydrophobic and antimicrobial ointments (eg, silver sulfadiazine cream) as well as frequent soaking in mild antiseptic solutions.[31] Nutritional support, fluid therapy, and pain management are often necessary. Feeding-tube placement should be considered in chelonians in order to facilitate oral fluid therapy and assisted feeding because the skin around the neck is often sloughed, making repeated restrain for orogastric gavage difficult. Recovery is usually prolonged and can take up to 4 to 6 months.

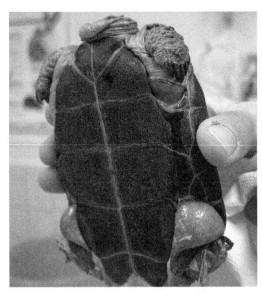

Fig. 7. Hypervitaminosis A in a turtle. Note the sloughing of the skin in the axillary and pre-femoral area. (*Courtesy of* J. Mayer, DVM, Athens, GA.)

Prevention

Avoid administration of vitamin A to herbivorous reptiles unless a vitamin A deficiency has been confirmed. In nonherbivorous reptiles, the repeated (>2–4 doses) administration of vitamin A parentally or orally at high dosages should be avoided because of the prolonged storage of vitamin A in the liver. Avoid excessive oral supplementation or feeding of excessive amounts of raw liver to semiaquatic turtles.

THIAMINE DEFICIENCY

Thiamine (vitamin B1) is a water-soluble vitamin synthesized by bacteria, fungi, and plants. Captive fish-eating reptiles, such as certain snakes species (eg, garter snakes [*Thamnophis spp*]), and semiaquatic turtles are most commonly affected if fish high in thiaminase is fed (eg, gold fish and fathead minnow [both are common feeder fish]). Feeder fish will become more thiamine deficient if they are fed frozen-thawed fish.[1] Thawing frozen fish slowly over several hours before feeding will lead to depletion of thiamine caused by enzymatic destruction by thiaminase, which is not destroyed during the freezing process.[1] Offering frozen-thawed vegetables, which contain phytothiaminases, has also been reported to potentially lead to thiamine deficiency in herbivorous reptiles, such as green iguanas (*Iguana iguana*).[1] Thiamine deficiency leading to neurologic deficits and mass mortalities has also been reported in wild American alligators (*Alligator mississippiensis*), eating thiaminase-positive fish (ie, gizzard shad [*Dorosoma cepedianum*]).[40]

Thiamine deficiency can also occur in insectivorous reptiles and has recently been reported in a breeding colony of *Anolis spp*[41] lizards. The suspected underlying cause of thiamine deficiency in this *Anolis* colony was the lack of thiamine in the multivitamin supplement caused by extensive storage of the supplement before use. Thiamine is a highly labile vitamin, which undergoes rapid deterioration under normal storage conditions.

Clinical Signs

Thiamine is vital in brain function, and a deficiency can cause degeneration of myelin sheaths of nerve fibers resulting in necrotizing encephalopathy and peripheral neuritis. Therefore, clinical signs include abnormal neurologic behavior manifesting as torticollis, opisthotonus, muscle tremors, incoordination, blindness, jaw gaping, and sudden death (**Fig. 8**).[1]

Diagnosis

The diagnosis of thiamine deficiency is usually made based on a combination of dietary history, clinical signs, and response to supplementation with thiamine. Thiamine deficiency may cause similar clinical signs as hypocalcemia; plasma calcium measurement, preferably plasma ionized calcium measurement, will aid in ruling out hypocalcaemia. Characteristic histopathologic findings consistent with thiamine deficiency include cerebral cortical necrosis and peripheral neuritis.[1,40]

Treatment

The administration of thiamine (50–100 mg/kg IM, SC, orally every 24 hours until clinical signs resolve) is recommended.[42] Alternatively, a vitamin B complex formulation that contains thiamine can be administered.

Prevention

Avoid feeding fish known to have high thiaminase levels, such as gold fish and fathead minnows. Proper storage and a rapid thawing process are critical to avoid thiamine depletion in frozen fish. Rapid thawing in 80°C (175°F) hot water for 5 minutes will lead to denaturation of thiaminase and prevent thiamine depletion during the thawing process.[1] Alternatively, frozen fish should be thawed in a refrigerator but not at room temperature to avoid activation of thiaminase. Routine supplementation of frozen-thawed fish with 20 mg of thiamine per kilogram of fish or the addition of small amounts of brewer's yeast is recommended.[1]

Reptile vitamin supplements should not be used beyond their expiration date because thiamin is a highly labile vitamin, and use of expired vitamin supplements has been shown to lead to thiamin deficiency in insectivorous *Anolis* lizards.

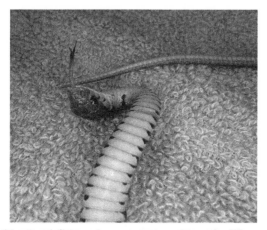

Fig. 8. Suspected thiamine deficiency in a common garter snake (*Thamnophis sirtalis*). This animal was fed exclusively on frozen feeder fish. (*Courtesy of* S. Barten, DVM, Mundelein, IL.)

HYPOVITAMINOSIS E

Vitamin E (tocopherol) deficiency is considered rare in captive reptiles but has been reported in American alligators, chelonians, green iguanas,[43] snakes,[44] veiled chameleons (*Chamaeleo calyptratus*),[45] and satanic leaf-tailed geckos (*Uroplatus phantasticus*).[46]

Vitamin E functions as an antioxidant and protects unsaturated fatty acids from oxidation. When deficient, the cellular components develop with abnormal structure, which affects the muscle, causing a nutritional myopathy. Additionally, in mammals, it affects the development of the fetus; abortions can result from deficiencies.[47]

The role of selenium deficiencies in the reported cases of hypovitaminosis E in reptiles remains unknown. Selenium, just like vitamin E, is part of biological antioxidant systems.[48] Selenium deficiencies in mammals result in similar clinical signs as vitamin E deficiencies.[2]

Myopathy secondary to suspected vitamin E/selenium deficiency has been suspected in a variety of insectivorous reptiles, including veiled chameleons and satanic leaf-tailed geckos.[45,46] The consistent histopathologic finding in these cases was generalized degenerative myopathy.

In aquatic carnivorous reptiles (eg, crocodilians, turtles), hypovitaminosis E has been associated with fish high in polyunsaturated fatty acids (eg, mackerel) stored under improper conditions, which allows for oxidization, leading to depletion of vitamin E.[1] Hypovitaminosis E in snakes has been associated with feeding obese laboratory rodents.[1]

Clinical Signs

In satanic leaf-tailed geckos with suspected hypovitaminosis E, the clinical signs included reduced appetite and activity as well as multifocal cutaneous red to white discolorations, which were characterized as dermal granulomas on histopathology.[46] In veiled chameleons with suspected hypovitaminosis E, the progressive inability to use the tongue, weakness, and circling were the main clinical signs.

Steatitis and fat necrosis is common in aquatic carnivorous reptiles (eg, crocodilians, turtles) and firm fatty subcutaneous nodules and are often seen in conjunction with anorexia.[2,49]

Diagnosis

The diagnosis of hypovitaminosis E is, in most cases, based on dietary history, physical examination findings, and histopathology. Tocopherol plasma or serum levels have not been used in the diagnosis of hypovitaminosis E. Limited reference values for plasma alpha-tocopherol levels are available.[48] Plasma alpha-tocopherol levels for captive and wild Eastern painted turtles (*Chrysemys picta picta*) ranged from 1.56 to 12.64 ug/mL.[48] Plasma levels in captive American alligators (*Alligator mississippiensis*) ranged from 2.49 to 6.15 ug/mL.[48]

Treatment

The reported parenteral doses of vitamin E for the treatment of suspected deficiencies vary and range from 1 to 50 U per kilogram of body weight administered by IM injection.[2,42]

Prevention

Diets should contain 20 to 80 IU/kg vitamin E based on dry matter.[1] Large amounts of vitamin E are contained in wheat germ and are often used to gut load insectivore prey.

However, most invertebrates contain sufficient amounts of vitamin E based on the recommendation of domestic mammalian carnivores (20–80 IU/kg dry matter).[11]

NUTRITIONAL SECONDARY HYPOTHYROIDISM

Iodine is considered a trace element essential for thyroid function serving as a component for thyroxine (T4) and triiodothyronine hormones.[2] These hormones, in turn, influence metabolism of all other nutrients and play a key role in stimulating carbohydrate and fat metabolism. In reptiles, ecdysis is controlled by the thyroid gland. Iodine is absorbed from the small intestine into the bloodstream. Approximately 30% of iodine goes to the thyroid, and the remainder is excreted via the kidneys in mammals as well as through sweat and feces. Storage in mammals occurs for 2 to 3 months in the thyroid follicles.

The thyroid gland in snakes is single or paired and is located ventral to the trachea just cranial to the heart.[50,51] In chelonians, the thyroid is a single gland and is located just cranial to the heart base.[51] In lizards, it is located cranial to the heart and has been reported to be single, bilobed, or paired, depending on the species.[52]

Goiter is the enlargement of the thyroid gland from various causes. Iodine deficiency is the most common cause for goiter in humans. In reptiles, dietary iodine deficiency and neoplasia of the thyroid gland have been reported.[50,53–57]

Deficiencies of thyroid hormones can occur because of insufficient dietary iodine intake or because of excessive intake of goitrogenic plant material, such as cruciferous plants (eg, broccoli, brussels sprouts, cauliflower, cabbage, cress, bok choy, kale).[2] These plants contain substances (goitrogens) that that lead to interference with the iodine uptake by the thyroid gland and subsequently cause a (nutritional secondary hypothyroidism) and goiter unless compensatory dietary iodine is ingested. When supplementing iodine, oversupplementation is a risk, with similar goiterogenic properties.

The reports of secondary dietary hypothyroidism, caused by iodine deficiency, in reptiles are limited and have mostly been reported in herbivorous lizards and chelonians.[53,54,58,59] However, most clinical case reports of hypothyroidism in tortoises do not fulfill the current standards of the diagnosis of insufficient function of the thyroid gland because an enlargement of the thyroid gland was not confirmed and a thyroid stimulation test was not performed. Therefore, several of the reported cases of hypothyroidism in chelonians in the literature might have been animals that suffered from euthyroid sick syndrome in which circulating thyroxin levels have been lower because of non-thyroidal systemic disorders.[2] A response to treatment with thyroxin does not confirm the diagnosis of hypothyroidism because increased metabolism, appetite, and activity are to be expected if thyroxin is supplemented in animals regardless if the thyroid is diseased or not.

Clinical Signs

In chelonians diagnosed with presumed or confirmed nutritional secondary hypothyroidism, edema of the neck, head, and forelimbs as well as decreased appetite and lethargy have been reported.[1,58,59] Reproductive failure, congenital malformations, prolonged gestation, skin problems, dwarfism, stunted growth, and reduced metabolic rates have been reported in cases of hypothyroidism in mammals; similar abnormalities may be seen in reptiles.[2,60]

Diagnosis

The diagnosis of hypothyroidism in reptiles should be made cautiously and should not rely on serum T4 levels alone. Thyroid function can only be adequately assessed by performing a thyroid stimulation test, which, to date, has not been reported in reptiles.

Low serum thyroxine levels can be caused by various physiological as well as thyroidal and non-thyroidal disease processes and do not necessarily reflect hypothyroidism. In reptiles, T4 levels are affected by the season and decrease during hibernation (brumation) and during fasting and increase following refeeding.[61] Serum thyroxine levels in African spurred tortoise (Centrochelys sulcata) have been reported to be lower (median 4 nmol/L [10th and 90th percentile: 2–9 nmol/L; n = 12])[62] than Galapagos tortoises (Geochelone nigra) (mean ± SD: 10.39 ± 18.72 nmol/L; n = 5)[63] and Aldabra tortoises (Aldabrachelys gigantea) (mean ± SD: 9 ± 3 nmol/L; n = 5).[59] However, the limited numbers of animals used in these studies limits the usefulness of these values as reference ranges. Therefore, interpretation of T4 levels in the absence of species-specific reference ranges should be performed cautiously.

In snakes, T4 levels range from 0.21 to 6.16 nmol/L.[64] Because normal thyroxin levels can be less than 1 nmol/L in snakes, using standard mammalian thyroxin tests is not recommended if hypothyroidism is suspected because these available tests are unlikely to be accurate at low levels.[64]

Given the lack of reference intervals, the influence of concurrent disease processes and the influence of environmental factors, the diagnosis of hypothyroidism caused by insufficient iodine intake or excessive intake of goitrogenic plants should be made cautiously.

Treatment

Iodine supplementation is rarely necessary if a balanced diet is fed. Given that over-supplementation can cause a similar clinical picture of a goiter, supplementation should be undertaken cautiously.[8] The levels of safe intake have not been described in reptiles; but given the variation in the metabolic rate caused by temperature, health status, seasonal and reproductive status, dietary intake, and natural history, the requirements likely vary significantly. When supplemented in reptiles, a multivitamin is likely sufficient. If supplementing iodine alone in deficient animals, the recommended dosages are 2 to 4 mg/kg daily for 2 to 3 weeks, then weekly.[42] Oral levothyroxine (0.02–0.025 mg/kg every 24–48 hours) has been administered in tortoises without obvious side effects.[54,59]

Prevention

The following has been suggested as the daily dietary iodine intake for reptiles: 0.3 µg/kg body weight.[1] Kelp (seaweed) is available commercially as powder or tablets and can be used as a source of iodine if the diet offered is iodine deficient. Avoid feeding goitrogenic plants in large quantities or on a routine basis.

DEHYDRATION

Dehydration in reptiles is often correlated with incorrect husbandry, particularly low humidity and lack of a temperature gradient in the enclosure. Further species that require a moving water source, such as the chameleon, are prone to dehydration if husbandry is incorrect. Variation in water needs occur with variations in natural history (ie, desert species vs tropical species). Many reptiles require supplemental soaking in captivity. Some will soak voluntarily in their habitat, whereas others will require forced soaking by the owner.

Clinical Signs

Signs of mild dehydration are subtle until the animal becomes more dehydrated. Improper ecdysis may be seen. Moderate to severely dehydrated animals are often depressed with sunken eyes (**Fig. 9**) and are anorexic, further contributing to their dehydrated state.

Diagnosis

The diagnosis of dehydration is based on the clinical signs. It can be assumed that most anorectic or chronically diseased reptiles are dehydrated. Skinfold testing may be reliable in lizards and snakes. Sunken eyes can also occur in cachexic reptiles and does not necessarily represent dehydration. Plasma electrolytes and uric acid and urea nitrogen might be helpful in the diagnosis of dehydration of reptiles but should be interpreted in conjunction with the clinical findings.

Treatment

To rehydrate, fluids can be given orally in mild cases; but usually for initial rehydration, the SC route is recommended. If dehydration is severe, then intraosseous, intravenous, or intracoelomic fluid administration should be performed. The recommended daily maintenance fluid requirements for most reptiles are 10 to 30 mL/kg. Fluids should be warmed to the specific preferred optimal temperature for each reptile patient.

Contrary to the common belief and historical recommendations, reptile plasma osmolality is similar or higher to that of mammalian or human plasma.[65–67] Therefore, the recommendation to dilute commercially balanced electrolyte solutions, to avoid the administration of hypertonic solution because of the presumed lower osmolality of reptiles' intercellular fluid, is not supported.[68,69] All reptile species investigated have similar or higher plasma osmolality compared with humans, dogs, and cats.

Plasma osmolality in bearded dragons is 295 ± 9.35 mOsm/kg[66] and 327 ± 3.3 mOsml/kg in green iguanas.[65] In corn snakes (*Pantherophis guttatus*), the mean plasma osmolality was higher, with 344.5 mmol/L (304.5–373.0 mOsm/kg).[66,67] Therefore, commercially available balanced electrolyte solutions (eg, lactated Ringer solution [272 mOsml/L], Normosol-R [295 mOsm/L] Plasmalyte-A [294 mOsm/L]) are

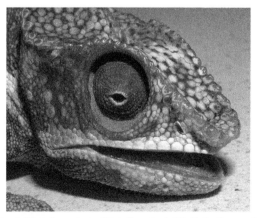

Fig. 9. Dehydrated panther chameleon (*Furcifer pardalis*). Note the sunken eyes. (*Courtesy of* S. Barten, DVM, Mundelein, IL.)

suitable for most cases. It needs to be considered that dehydration can lead to an increase in plasma osmolality; therefore, reference values established in healthy and hydrated reptiles should be used cautiously.

Soaking is also an effective method of treating dehydrated reptiles, particularly for cases of mild dehydration of if dehydrated reptiles cannot be hospitalized for parenteral fluid therapy. Care should be taken to avoid drowning in debilitated animals. Therefore, water levels should be shallow and supervision should be provided.

Prevention

Provide adequate temperature gradients within the enclosure and a day-night temperature fluctuation, as appropriate for the species. Ensure appropriate humidity and access to water, depending on the species; consider regular soaking.

OBESITY

Obesity is a concern in captive reptiles when energy intake is greater than energy requirements. Free access to food can cause overconsumption with a lack of expenditure of energy. Further, food items high in fat will promote obesity. In general, larva forms of insects contain significantly more fat than adults (eg, worms vs beetles). For example, beetles of the superworm (*Zophobas morio*) and mealworm (*Tenebrio molitor*) contain more protein and one-half to one-third of the fat content as the larva of the same species while having similar mineral contents.[13] In contrast, earlier stages (nymphs) of cockroaches as well as crickets usually are higher in protein and lower in fat compared with larger (older) animals.[11,13]

A lack of hibernation in captivity has been proposed as a cause of obesity in some captive reptiles.

Clinical Signs

Excessive intracoelomic fat storage may lead to coelomic distension (**Fig. 10**A). This condition should be differentiated from disease processes, such as ascites or tympany, or from physiologic hyperinflation of the lungs and air sacs in certain lizard species during handling. Fat stores in reptiles, as in other animals, can be subcutaneous (see **Fig. 10**B, C), intracoelomic, and parenchymal.[2] Obese reptiles often have increased fat over the vertebral column, and certain gecko species store fat in their tail (eg, leopard geckos). Fatty infiltration of parenchymal organs, such as the liver, may occur (ie, hepatic lipidosis).

Diagnosis

Diagnosis is based on the physical examination and history.

Treatment and Prevention

Significant variation in metabolic rate is seen with changes in reproductive status, body mass, seasonal cycles and light cycles, diet, and many other factors. Essentially very little is known in the real-life needs for a given species in captivity, and weights should be monitored closely at home to ensure correct feeding amounts as well as for weight loss as a sign of disease processes. Overfeeding as well as maintaining reptiles in small enclosures which promote a sedentary lifestyle should be avoided.

Just as for any species, remedying the problem requires both a dietary change and increasing exercise. Carnivores should be fed very lean prey. Herbivores should have

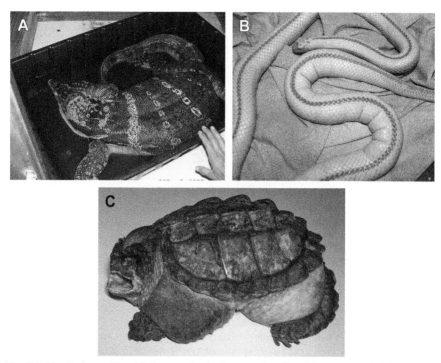

Fig. 10. Obesity in reptiles. (*A*) Severe obesity in a monitor lizard (*Varanus* spp). (*B*) Excessive subcutaneous fat in an obese California kingsnake (*Lampropeltis getula californiae*). (*C*) Morbidly obese common snapping turtle (*Chelydra serpentine*) with excessive subcutaneous fat. (*Courtesy of* [*A*] Special Species Health Service, School of Veterinary Medicine, University of Wisconsin; and [*B, C*] S. Barten, DVM, Mundelein, IL.)

an increase in dietary fiber. A thorough work-up to rule out concurrent health problems before attempting weight loss is recommended.

ANOREXIA AND CACHEXIA

Anorexia leading to starvation and cachexia can be from a variety of causes; in particular, incorrect husbandry should be considered. Inappropriate food items, stress (eg, caused by overcrowding, frequent handling, lack of hiding places), and inappropriate environmental temperatures are common environmental causes for anorexia in captive reptiles. Many female gravid reptiles will show physiologic temporary anorexia. Reduced food and consequently caloric intake will lead to a loss of muscle and fat tissue and will lead to dehydration unless water intake is maintained. Mobilization of body fat can lead to increased accumulation of fat within the hepatocytes, leading to hepatic lipidosis, which may further contribute to anorexia.

Clinical Signs

Anorexic reptiles may present without any clinical abnormalities; but with prolonged anorexia and/or underlying disease processes, loss of muscle and body fat is evident by prominent vertebral processes and iliac crests (**Fig. 11**). The eyes may be sunken in cachexic lizards and chelonians. Frequently, dehydration can be noted on the physical

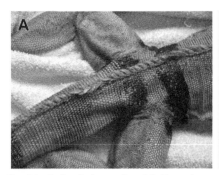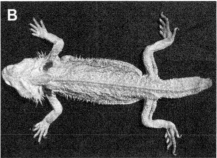

Fig. 11. Cachexia in reptiles. (*A*) Green iguana (*Iguana iguana*). Note the loss of muscle mass and the prominent pelvic bones. (*B*) Severely cachexic and dehydrated bearded dragon (*Pogona vitticeps*). Note the complete lack of muscle mass. (*Courtesy of* M. Pinkerton, DVM, DACVP, Madison, WI.)

examination. Depending on the underlying cause, affected reptiles can be bright and alert or lethargic and depressed.

Diagnosis

A thorough review of the husbandry and diet is critical because of the common occurrence of environmental causes leading to anorexia and cachexia in reptiles. Ruling out infectious and noninfectious causes should be performed as appropriate for the species. Clinical pathology and diagnostic imaging should be used to establish a diagnosis if an environmental cause has been ruled out. Assessment of the liver by computed tomography, ultrasonography or laparoscopy, and tissue biopsy should be considered in order to rule out hepatic lipidosis.[70]

Treatment

Dehydration, which is present in most anorexic and cachexic reptiles, should be corrected before the initiation of nutritional support. Providing general guidelines for nutritional support of anorexic and cachexic reptiles is challenging because of the diversity among common captive reptiles, and caloric requirements depend on age and underlying disease processes.

Enteral feeding of anorexic reptiles can be accomplished by orogastric gavage using ball-tipped catheters or flexible feeding tubes. Single or repeated feedings can be performed in most lizards and snakes using orogastric gavage and manual restraint. In chelonians, in particular tortoises, proper restraint for orogastric gavage might be challenging without sedation; repeated restraint and gavage is likely stressful. Therefore, placement of an esophageal feeding tube should be strongly considered in order to allow the administration of nutrients but also medications via the enteral route (**Fig. 12**). Volume recommendations for orogastric administration of enteral feeding formulas range between 2% and 10% of body weight.[1] Energy density of fiber content of the used formula will affect the amount being administered. It is recommended to initially administer smaller amounts of feeding formula, and monitor for fecal output, before administering larger amounts of feeding formula. A variety of enteral feeding formulas are available for veterinary use and should be chosen based on the reptile species' dietary requirements. Overfeeding of starved reptiles can lead to a condition called refeeding syndrome, which is characterized by life-threatening hypokalemia and hypophosphatemia.[2] Therefore, too rapid an increase in the amount of food provided to starved reptiles should be avoided; plasma electrolyte, phosphorus, and glucose levels should be monitored.[2]

SOFT FECES AND DIARRHEA

Fecal consistency varies physiologically between reptile species and mainly depends on their diet. It is, therefore, important to be aware of the species-specific normal fecal consistency in order to avoid misinterpretation of normal fecal consistency as diarrhea. Soft feces or diarrhea is common, particularly in herbivore reptiles being fed an inappropriate diet low in fiber and/or high in fermentable simple carbohydrates (eg, fruits). Environmental factors, such as low temperatures, lead to decreased gastrointestinal motility and disturbances.[71] Endoparasites are a very common for soft feces and diarrhea in captive reptiles. Other infectious causes that are much less common in captive reptiles include viral, fungal, and bacterial organisms.[71]

Clinical Signs

Herbivorous reptiles with diarrhea caused by an inappropriate diet might show no other clinical signs or may show unspecific clinical signs, such as lethargy, reduced food intake, or dehydration. Tympany and other gastrointestinal disorders might be present.[70]

Diagnosis

The diagnosis in most cases can be made based on a thorough review of the husbandry and, in particular, the diet. Physical examination and fecal parasitology (direct fecal wet mount, fecal flotation) should be performed to rule out nondietary causes of diarrhea. Diagnostic imaging, clinical pathology, and endoscopy of the gastrointestinal tract should be considered if deemed appropriate to rule out nondietary causes.[70]

Treatment and Prevention

Treatment of diarrhea in reptiles depends on the underlying cause. High numbers of endoparasites should be treated, even though they might not be the primary cause. Dehydration and environmental problems, such as inadequate husbandry, need to be corrected. Appropriate amounts of fiber should be fed; fermentable sugars contained in fruits should be avoided, unless appropriate for the reptile species.

CONSTIPATION

The causes of irregular defecation, fecal retention, and constipation are multiple. A lack of fiber or inadequate exercise are common causes of constipation. Chronic dehydration caused by inappropriate environmental temperature (lack of temperature gradient, lack of day/night temperature difference); insufficient or inappropriate water sources; low humidity; long-haired prey; hard-shelled insect prey; or ingestion of indigestible substrate, such as sand, gravel, or bark have been reported.[52,72] Metabolic causes, such as hypocalcemia, should be considered. Differentials for constipation unrelated to diet or husbandry should include chronic systemic disease (eg, kidney disease, anemia) and intestinal neoplasia. Extramural causes include kidney enlargement caused by nephritis in lizards, uroliths, cloacoliths, neoplasia, abscesses, and narrowed pelvic canal in lizards and chelonians caused by healed fractures or reproductive disease and presence of eggs.[72,73]

Clinical Signs

Lack or reduced fecal output with or without straining is common in reptiles suffering from constipation. Depending on the severity of constipation, anorexia, dehydration, and lethargy may be noted. Coelomic palpation in lizards and snakes may reveal excessive amounts of ingesta and fecal material in the large intestine.

Diagnosis

Radiographs or computed tomography are usually diagnostic. Contrast radiography can be used to rule out obstructive conditions.[70] Plasma biochemistry will help to rule out metabolic causes (see NSHP).

Treatment and Prevention

The primary focus of therapy should be to correct the identified underlying cause, such as insufficient fiber content or environmental temperatures that are too low. Correct the dehydration; optimize humidity and environmental temperatures; correct

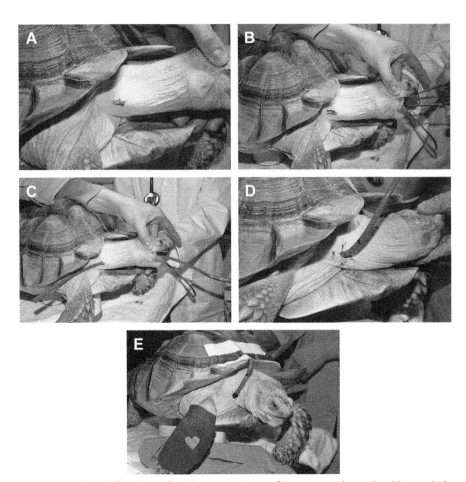

Fig. 12. Esophageal feeding tube placement in an African spurred tortoise (*Centrochelys sulcata*).

metabolic causes; the increase fiber content in the diet of herbivorous or omnivorous reptiles; and increase enclosure to provide more exercise. Enteral fluid therapy is considered the most effective method for relief of constipation by rehydrating fecal material and ingesta and promoting gastrointestinal motility. Lizards and snakes can be administered fluids via gastric gavage. However, in chelonians, particularly tortoises, repeated administration of fluids via stomach gavage is stressful and labor intensive. Instead, consider placement of an esophageal feeding tube to allow easy and repeated enteral fluid and drug administration (**Fig. 12**).

Enemas or cloacal washes are a very effective way to relieve rectal constipation and should be considered particularly in lizards. Use warmed tap water and a red-rubber catheter or ball-tipped gavage needle. The risk of entering the urinary bladder instead of the rectum is high in lizards, which have a functional bladder. However, bearded dragons do not have a functional bladder; therefore, enemas are very effective. Great care should be taken to avoid iatrogenic damage, and therefore careful placement of the tube or catheter after lubrication should be performed. Daily soaking in warm tap water may also aid in rehydration and promotes defecation in many reptiles.

Medical therapy has been suggested for treatment of constipation of reptiles and should be considered if enteral fluid therapy and correction of environmental causes have not resolved the constipation or it has reoccurred. Psyllium is an indigestive fiber and acts as a bulk laxative. Sufficient hydration and water intake should be ensured before administration. Prevention of constipation should focus on an appropriate diet and husbandry.

REFERENCES

1. Calvert I. Nutritional problems. In: Girling SJ, Raiti P, editors. BSAVA manual of reptiles. Glouchester (United Kingdom): British Small Animal Veterinary Association; 2004. p. 289–308.
2. Donoghue S. Nutrition. In: Mader DR, editor. Reptile medicine and surgery. St Louis (MO): Elsevier; 2006. p. 251–98.
3. Klaphake E. A fresh look at metabolic bone diseases in reptiles and amphibians. Vet Clin North Am Exot Anim Pract 2010;13(3):375–92.
4. Ferguson GW, Gehrmann WH, Karsten KB, et al. Do panther chameleons bask to regulate endogenous vitamin D3 production? Physiol Biochem Zool 2003; 76(1):52–9.
5. Acierno MJ, Mitchell MA, Roundtree MK, et al. Effects of ultraviolet radiation on 25-hydroxyvitamin D3 synthesis in red-eared slider turtles (Trachemys scripta elegans). Am J Vet Res 2006;67(12):2046–9.
6. Acierno MJ, Mitchell MA, Zachariah TT, et al. Effects of ultraviolet radiation on plasma 25-hydroxyvitamin D3 concentrations in corn snakes (Elaphe guttata). Am J Vet Res 2008;69(2):294–7.
7. Hedley J, Eatwell K. The effects of UV light on calcium metabolism in ball pythons (*Python regius*). Vet Rec 2013;173(14):345.
8. Selleri P, Di Girolamo N. Plasma 25-hydroxyvitamin D(3) concentrations in Hermann's tortoises (Testudo hermanni) exposed to natural sunlight and two artificial ultraviolet radiation sources. Am J Vet Res 2012;73(11):1781–6.
9. Oonincx DG, Stevens Y, van den Borne JJ, et al. Effects of vitamin D3 supplementation and UVb exposure on the growth and plasma concentration of vitamin D3 metabolites in juvenile bearded dragons (Pogona vitticeps). Comp Biochem Physiol B Biochem Mol Biol 2010;156(2):122–8.

10. Gramanzini M, Di Girolamo N, Gargiulo S, et al. Assessment of dual-energy x-ray absorptiometry for use in evaluating the effects of dietary and environmental management on Hermann's tortoises (Testudo hermanni). Am J Vet Res 2013; 74(6):918–24.

11. Barker D, Fitzpatrick MP, Dierenfeld ES. Nutrient composition of selected whole invertebrates. Zoo Biol 1998;17(2):123–34.

12. Dierenfeld E, King J. Digestibility and mineral availability of Phoenix worms, Hermetia illucens, ingested by mountain chicken frogs, Leptodactylus fallax. J Herpetol Med Surg 2008;18(3/4):100–5.

13. Oonincx D, Dierenfeld ES. An investigation into the chemical composition of alternative invertebrate prey. Zoo Biol 2012;31(1):40–54.

14. Dennis PM, Bennett RA, Harr KE, et al. Plasma concentration of ionized calcium in healthy iguanas. J Am Vet Med Assoc 2001;219(3):326–8.

15. Eatwell K. Plasma concentrations of 25-hydroxycholecalciferol in 22 captive tortoises (Testudo species). Vet Rec 2008;162(11):342–5.

16. Lauten SD, Cox NR, Brawner WR Jr, et al. Use of dual energy x-ray absorptiometry for noninvasive body composition measurements in clinically normal dogs. Am J Vet Res 2001;62(8):1295–301.

17. Zotti A, Selleri P, Carnier P, et al. Relationship between metabolic bone disease and bone mineral density measured by dual-energy X-ray absorptiometry in the green iguana (Iguana iguana). Vet Radiol Ultrasound 2004;45(1):10–6.

18. Greer LL, Daniel GB, Bartges JW, et al. Evaluation of bone mineral density in the healthy green iguana, Iguana iguana: correlation of dual energy x-ray absorptiometry and radiology. J Herpetol Med Surg 2006;16(1):4–8.

19. Finke MD. Gut loading to enhance the nutrient content of insects as food for reptiles: a mathematical approach. Zoo Biol 2003;22(2):147–62.

20. Wallach JD. Hypervitaminosis D in green iguanas. J Am Vet Med Assoc 1966; 149(7):912–4.

21. Fledelius B, Jorgensen GW, Jensen HE, et al. Influence of the calcium content of the diet offered to leopard tortoises (Geochelone pardalis). Vet Rec 2005;156(26):831–5.

22. Burger RM, Gehrmann WH, Ferguson GW. Evaluation of UVB reduction by materials commonly used in reptile husbandry. Zoo Biol 2007;26(5):417–23.

23. Hand MS, Lewis LD. Small animal clinical nutrition. Topeka (KS): Mark Morris Institute; 2010.

24. Black GB. Avian Nurition. Minneapolis (MN): Avian Publications; 2006.

25. Raila J, Schuhmacher A, Gropp J, et al. Selective absorption of carotenoids in the common green iguana (Iguana iguana). Comp Biochem Physiol A Mol Integr Physiol 2002;132(2):513–8.

26. Koelle P, Wiedemann A, Kienzle E. Vitamin A in plasma of reptiles. Proceedings of the Association of Reptile and Amphibian Veterinarians. South Padre Island (TX): Association of Reptile and Amphibian Veterinarians; 2010. p. 4–6.

27. Bausch J, Rietz P. Method for the assessment of vitamin A liver stores. Acta Vitaminol Enzymol 1977;31(1–5):99–112.

28. San-Jose LM, Granado-Lorencio F, Fitze PS. Vitamin E, vitamin A, and carotenoids in male common lizard tissues. Herpetologica 2012;68(1):88–99.

29. Boyer TH. Hypovitaminosis A and hypervitaminosis A. In: Mader DR, editor. Reptile medicine and surgery. St Louis (MO): Elsevier; 2006. p. 831–5.

30. Elkan E, Zwart P. The ocular disease of young terrapins caused by vitamin A deficiency. Pathol Vet 1967;4(3):201–22.

31. Stahl SJ. Hypovitaminosis A. In: Mayer J, Donnelly TM, editors. Clinical veterinary advisor: birds and exotic pets. St Louis (MO): Elsevier; 2013. p. 108–10.

32. Ariel E, Ladds PW, Buenviaje GN. Concurrent gout and suspected hypovitaminosis A in crocodile hatchlings. Aust Vet J 1997;75(4):247–9.
33. Ferguson GW, Jones JR, Gehrmann WH, et al. Indoor husbandry of the panther chameleon Chamaeleo Furcifer pardalis: effects of dietary vitamins A and D and ultraviolet irradiation on pathology and life-history traits. Zoo Biol 1996;15(3): 279–99.
34. Sleeman JM, Brown J, Steffen D, et al. Relationships among aural abscesses, organochlorine compounds, and vitamin a in free-ranging Eastern box turtles (Terrapene carolina carolina). J Wildl Dis 2008;44(4):922–9.
35. Raphael BL, Klemens MW, Moehlman P, et al. Blood values in free-ranging pancake tortoises (Malacochersus-Tornieri). J Zoo Wildl Med 1994;25(1):63–7.
36. Anderson MD, et al. Hypervitaminosis A in the young pig. J Anim Sci 1966;25(4): 1123–7.
37. Dobson KJ. Osteodystrophy associated with hypervitaminosis a in growing pigs. Aust Vet J 1969;45(12):570–3.
38. Ogilvy V, Fidgett AL, Preziosi RF. Differences in carotenoid accumulation among three feeder-cricket species: implications for carotenoid delivery to captive insectivores. Zoo Biol 2012;31(4):470–8.
39. Mettler F, Palmer D, Rubel A, et al. High incidence of parakeratosis with detachment of skin epithelium among tortoises. Zurich (Switzerland); 33 cases in 4 years; possible role of vitamin injections [Gehauft auftretende Falle von Parakeratose mit Epithelablosung der Haut bei Landschildkroten]. Erkrankungen der Zootiere. Verhandlungsbericht des XXIV. Internationalen Symposiums uber die Erkrankungen der Zootiere vom 19. Mai bis 23. Mai 1982 in Veszprem, 1982.
40. Honeyfield DC, Ross JP, Carbonneau DA, et al. Pathology, physiologic parameters, tissue contaminants, and tissue thiamine in morbid and healthy central Florida adult American alligators (Alligator mississippiensis). J Wildl Dis 2008;44(2):280–94.
41. Feldman SH, Formica M, Brodie ED. Opisthotonus, torticollis and mortality in a breeding colony of Anolis sp lizards thiamine deficiency. Lab Anim (NY) 2011; 40(4):107–8.
42. Carpenter JW, Klaphake E, Gibbons PM. Reptile formulary and laboratory normals. In: Mader DR, Divers SJ, editors. Current therapy in reptile medicine & surgery. St Louis (MO): Saunders-Elsevier; 2014. p. 393.
43. Farnsworth RJ, Brannian RE, Fletcher KC, et al. A vitamin E-selenium responsive condition in a green iguana. J Zoo Wildl Med 1986;17(1):42–3.
44. Langham RF, Zydeck FA, Bennett RR. Steatitis in a captive Marcy garter snake. J Am Vet Med Assoc 1971;159(5):640–1.
45. Cole G, Rao DB, Steinberg H, et al. Suspected vitamin E and selenium deficiency in a veiled chameleon (Chamaeleo calyptratus). J Herpetol Med Surg 2008; 18(3/4):113–6.
46. Gabor LJ. Nutritional degenerative myopathy in a population of captive bred Uroplatus phantasticus (satanic leaf-tailed geckoes). J Vet Diagn Invest 2005; 17(1):71–3.
47. Hall JE. Guyton and Hall textbook of medical physiology. 12th edition. Philladelphia: Saunders-Elsevier; 2010.
48. Dierenfeld ES. Vitamin-E-deficiency in zoo reptiles, birds, and ungulates. J Zoo Wildl Med 1989;20(1):3–11.
49. Larsen RE, Buergelt C, Cardeilhac PT, et al. Steatitis and fat necrosis in captive alligators. J Am Vet Med Assoc 1983;183(11):1202–4.

50. Topper MJ, Latimer KS, McManamon R, et al. Colloid goiter in an Eastern diamondback rattlesnake (*Crotalus-adamanteus*). Vet Pathol 1994;31(3):380–2.

51. O'Malley B. Clinical anatomy and physiology of exotic species. St. Louis (MO): Saunders-Elsevier; 2005.

52. Barten SL. Lizards. In: Mader DR, editor. Reptile medicine and surgery. St Louis (MO): Elsevier; 2006. p. 59–77, 683–95.

53. Janos G. Goitre in an Egyptian tortoise (*Testudo kleinmanni*). Magy Allatorvosok Lapja 2007;129(8):490–3.

54. Norton TM, Jacobson ER, Caligiuri R, et al. Medical-management of a Galapagos tortoise (*Geochelone-Elephantopus*) with hypothyroidism. J Zoo Wildl Med 1989;20(2):212–6.

55. Boyer TH, Wallack S, Bettencourt A, et al. Hyperthyroidism in a leopard gecko (*Eublepharis macularius*) and radioiodine (*I-131*) treatment. South Padre Island (TX): Proceeding Association of Reptilian and Amphibian Veterinarians; 2010. p. 53.

56. Gal J, Csiko G, Pasztor I, et al. First description of papillary carcinoma in the thyroid gland of a red-eared slider (Trachemys scripta elegans). Acta Vet Hung 2010;58(1):69–73.

57. Hadfield CA, Clayton LA, Clancy MM, et al. Proliferative thyroid lesions in three diplodactylid geckos: Nephrurus amyae, Nephrurus levis, and Oedura marmorata. J Zoo Wildl Med 2012;43(1):131–40.

58. Frye FL, Dutra FR. Hypothyroidism in turtles and tortoises. Vet Med Small Anim Clin 1974;69(8):990–3.

59. Franco KH, Hoover JP. Levothyroxine as a treatment for presumed hypothyroidism in an adult male African spurred tortoise (Centrochelys [formerly Geochelone] sulcata). J Herpetol Med Surg 2009;19(2):42–4.

60. Denver RJ, Licht P. Dependence of body growth on thyroid-activity in turtles. J Exp Zool 1991;258(1):48–59.

61. Kohel KA, MacKenzie DS, Rostal DC, et al. Seasonality in plasma thyroxine in the desert tortoise, Gopherus agassizii. Gen Comp Endocrinol 2001;121(2):214–22.

62. Franco KH, Famini DJ, Hoover JP, et al. Serum thyroid hormone values for African spurred tortoises (Centrochelys [formerly Geochelone] sulcata). J Herpetol Med Surg 2009;19(2):47–9.

63. DiGesualdo CL, West G, Brown TR, et al. Determining normal thyroid hormone status in Galapagos tortoises (Geochelone elephantopus) suspected of hypothyroidism. Proceedings American Association of Zoo Veterinarians. San Diego (CA): American Association of Zoo Veterinarians; 2004. p. 550–1.

64. Greenacre CB, Young DW, Behrend EN, et al. Validation of a novel high-sensitivity radioimmunoassay procedure for measurement of total thyroxine concentration in psittacine birds and snakes. Am J Vet Res 2001;62(11):1750–4.

65. Fitzsimons JT, Kaufman S. Cellular and extracellular dehydration, and angiotensin as stimuli to drinking in the common iguana Iguana iguana. J Physiol 1977;265(2):443–63.

66. Dallwig RK, Mitchell MA, Acierno MJ. Determination of plasma osmolality and agreement between measured and calculated values in healthy adult bearded dragons (*Pogona vitticeps*). J Herpetol Med Surg 2010;20(2–3):69–73.

67. Guzman DS, Mitchell MA, Acierno M. Determination of plasma osmolality and agreement between measured and calculated values in captive male corn snakes (*Pantherophis* [*Elaphe*] *guttatus guttatus*). J Herpetol Med Surg 2011; 21(1):16–9.

68. Davis RR, Klingenberg RJ. Therapeutics and medication. In: Girling SJ, Raiti P, editors. BSAVA manual of reptiles. Gloucester (United Kingdom): British Small Animal Veterinary Association; 2004. p. 115–30.
69. Orosz SE. Critical care nutrition for exotic animals. J Exot Pet Med 2013;22(2): 163–77.
70. Mans C. Clinical update on diagnosis and management of disorders of the digestive system of reptiles. J Exot Pet Med 2013;22(2):141–62.
71. Hnizdo J, Pantchev N. Medical care of turtles & tortoises. Frankfurt (Germany): Edition Chimaira; 2011.
72. McArthur S, McLellan L, Brown S. Gastrointestinal system. In: Girling SJ, Raiti P, editors. BSAVA manual of reptiles. Gloucester (United Kingdom): British Small Animal Veterinary Association; 2004. p. 210–29.
73. Knotkova Z, Knotek Z, Hajkova P, et al. Renal disease haemogram and plasma biochemistry in green iguana. Acta Vet Brno 2002;71(3):333–40.

Clinical Avian Nutrition

Susan E. Orosz, PhD, DVM, DABVP (Avian), DECZM (Avian)

KEYWORDS

- Nutrition • Psittacine • Avian • Diet • Foraging • Minerals • Vitamins • Proteins

KEY POINTS

- Companion psittacine birds eat plant-based foods; primarily grains (cockatiels and budgerigars), fruiting bodies (many of the macaws), and nectar (lories and lorikeets).
- Birds in the wild do not necessarily select adequate diets nutritionally, and companion birds do not do as well when self-selecting diets, which suggests that balanced diets are needed to improve general health in companion birds.
- Seed-only diets are deficient in fat-soluble vitamins, major minerals (Ca, PO_4, Na, Mn, Zn, Fe, I, Se), often high in fats, and the amino acids are unbalanced.
- A nutritional history is important to determine whether the avian patient is in balance nutritionally.
- The diet should contain a large percentage of balanced foods that are often provided as formulated foods, followed by vegetables, nuts, and other protein sources, and a small serving of fruits (true berries preferred).
- Foraging is important for companion birds to express their natural behaviors.

NUTRITIONAL NEEDS

Veterinarians and veterinary technicians are commonly asked questions relating to avian nutrition in the examination room. Veterinarians need to make clinical judgments regarding nutrition in avian patients including those with various diseases. However, nutrition is often only touched on in the veterinary curriculum and birds are rarely discussed. This article focuses on what veterinarians and technicians need to know to complement and improve the quality of their care for companion avian patients with well birds. Information is also provided to enhance the discussion of nutrition with the client in the examination room.

WHAT ARE THE NUTRITIONAL FEEDING STRATEGIES OF PSITTACINE BIRDS?

The types of foodstuffs consumed in the wild are used as a tool to classify groups of animals for helping to determine the nutritional requirements. In general, the birds

Conflict of Interest: The author is a consultant for Lafeber Company.
Bird & Exotic Pet Wellness Center, 5166 Monroe Street, Toledo, OH 43623, USA
E-mail address: drsusanorosz@aol.com

within the order Psittaciformes are considered to consume plant-based foodstuffs and are classified as florivores. Within this category, further subclassifications can be made, including granivory (eg, budgies and cockatiels), frugivory (many of the macaws; eg, green-winged macaw), and nectarivory (eg, lorikeets and lories). However, many psittacine birds cross these artificial lines and consume a larger variety of foodstuffs. An example is the scarlet macaw. This macaw is classified as a frugivorous-granivorous psittacine. In addition to the basic classification based on general foods eaten, ingredients consumed vary over time depending on nutrient availability, sex of the bird, and age.[1] However, there are some species that have a limited diet, like the glossy black cockatoo (*Calyptorhyncus lathami*), which feeds almost exclusively on the seeds from a single species of tree in its native environment (**Table 1**).

NUTRIENT REQUIREMENTS

Nutrients are defined as the components in the diet that provide the energy to maintain life and provide the precursors for the synthesis of the structural and functional macromolecules. The macromolecules provide most of the diet and include lipids, proteins, carbohydrates, and water. Micronutrients are the smaller nutrients of the diet and include vitamins and minerals. Essential nutrients are required for optimal health. They may be needed for metabolism and may not be synthesized in sufficient amounts

Table 1
Feeding strategies and common diet ingredients of wild psittacine birds

Species Name	Feeding Strategy	Common Diet Ingredients	Time Spent Feeding (h/d)
Blue and gold macaw (*Ara araraunda*)	Florivore	Seeds, fruits, nuts	NR
Military macaw (*Ara militaris*)	Florivore	Seeds, nuts, berries, fruits	NR
Green-winged macaw (*Ara chloroptera*)	Frugivore	Fruits (*Hymenaea*), palm nuts, seeds	NR
Orange-winged Amazon (*Amazona amazonica*)	Frugivore	Fruit (85% from palm fruit)	NR
Scarlet macaw (*Ara macao*)	Frugivore-granivore	Fruits, nuts, bark, leaves, shoots	NR
Budgerigar (*Melopsittacus undulatus*)	Granivore	Seeds	NR
Cockatiel (*Nymphicus hollandicus*)	Granivore	Seeds (prefers soft, young, overmature, hard seeds)	3
Hyacinth macaw (*Anodorhynchus hyacinthinus*)	Granivore	Palm nuts (50% lipid content)	NR
Sulphur-crested cockatoo (*Cacatua galerita*)	Omnivore	Seeds (primarily sunflower), grubs, rhizomes	NR

Abbreviation: NR, Not reported.
Adapted from Koutsos EA, Matson KD, Klasing KC. Nutrition of birds in the order Psittaciformes: a review. J Avian Med Surg 2001;15:257–75.

to meet the metabolic demands. The quantity needed is described as the requirement of the particular nutrient. The qualitative and quantitative components of the nutrient requirements are well known in some of the domestic galliforms, an order of birds that includes chickens, turkeys, and Japanese quail as well as domestic ducks. The essential nutrients are required in similar proportions with these species and for this reason have been used as a model for psittacines. Energy is a property that nutrients possess and is not a chemically definable nutrient. However, a variety of nutrients, when oxidized during metabolism of foodstuffs, results in the production of energy.

The physiology of a particular species determines its nutrient requirements. Requirements are determined for 3 physiologic states: basal, maintenance, and total. The basal requirements are those needed to maintain basic life functions; that is, those needed to replace losses inherent in being alive. The maintenance requirement is the amount of nutrients needed for basal functions, including the activity of finding and consuming food, interacting with other animals, and maintaining body temperature. The total energy requirement is the combination of all requirements for life and its stages, including growth, reproduction, and molt.

It is important to understand the principles behind how nutrient requirements are determined, particularly with companion species of birds. Few nutrient requirements have been studied scientifically, so nutrient requirements are often based on the best guess from those derived from galliforms. Even in these species, requirements have been determined using 2 methods: empirically and by calculations based on factorial summation of specific needs. With empirically based recommendations, experimental diets with graded nutrient levels are fed to a particular species. The minimal level that optimizes the birds' health and performance is considered the level requirement.

One example that has been cited concerns feeding groups of galliform chicks increasing levels of methionine. With this nutrient, their growth rate increases linearly and the point at which the growth rate does not increase with increasing levels of methionine is empirically determined to be the requirement level of this nutrient. Often the line between levels that are deficient and those that are adequate is not sharp and follows the law of diminishing returns.

Factorial calculations involve adding together various requirements to determine the needs for a particular situation. For example, the requirement of methionine during the egg-laying stage has been determined by adding the maintenance requirement in the egg (as determined from the amounts of this nutrient found in the egg) to the amount needed by the reproductive tract during the egg-laying period. This factorial method of calculating a nutrient requirement is often used for determining energy requirements, amino acid requirements, and necessary calcium levels during lay, for example. This technique can be very accurate as long as the information on which it is based is also accurate.

The problem with companion birds is that these requirements are often not well established. The other problem is that the efficiency of absorption of nutrients, especially for life stages, may not be accurate. Varying absorption efficiencies may thus throw off the calculations. Both methods, empirical and factorial summation, have been combined to formulate the requirements for galliforms and ducks and published as the US National Academy of Sciences report.[2] These values represent the nutrient requirements under optimal conditions for these species. Particularly in companion birds, a margin of safety is added to these values derived from galliforms and provides the best educated guess for adequate nutrition. The Association of Avian Veterinarians (AAV) worked with a panel of experts in diverse areas of avian nutrition to provide general recommendations for psittacines and passerines. These values were the best collective guess to start the discussion on nutrient requirements in these groups of companion birds.[3] Avian clinicians realize that individual species have differing needs based on their clinical impressions and the natural behaviors of their wild cousins. Additional concerns about feeding whole-food diets in mammals and providing foods that allow companion birds to show their natural foraging behaviors is adding to a better understanding of their nutritional needs.

Birds in the wild do not necessarily select adequate diets nutritionally, although they seem to be able to balance their energy needs, amino acids, and calcium, but not their other requirements.[1] Birds in captivity do not seem to select appropriately either. A self-selected diet in African gray parrots (*Psittacus erithacus*)[4] resulted in a diet that was deficient in a total of 12 dietary components consisting of vitamins, minerals, and amino acids. **Table 2** shows the suggested requirements of psittacines and passerines.

NUTRITIONAL HISTORY

A nutritional history should be taken from the client on the initial presentation of the avian patient. It should be also taken with each yearly examination because what clients admit they feed changes over time. During this history-taking process, it is important to let owners talk and give them the opportunity to explain what they are doing. This opportunity is important in the flow of the examination time period before offering constructive information to improve the quality of nutritional care. More information is gained that way. Often, the veterinary technician obtains the nutritional history along with the history relevant to the patient for this particular visit. The veterinarian may then review the patient history and ask specific questions or just ask the client to review some of the information. There can be significant differences in the information obtained from some clients by the technician and what the client tells the veterinarian.

As with other veterinary problems, what clients hear, what they remember, and what was discussed are often different. That is why going over the information by the technician and the avian veterinarian can prove helpful. Then, reviewing what the patient is consuming, each year, provides additional information on what was understood and followed from preceding visits.

It is important to determine the species, age of the patient, or numbers of birds in the flock; the use of the patient (ie, is this a breeding bird or a companion?); what the bird is offered at each meal; and how often the bird is fed in a day. Is it in a cage with another bird(s)?

It is important to establish what the patient eats each day and how much of each food item it eats. All of this information needs to be determined and recorded. The variety of foods offered per day helps determine whether there is a smorgasbord effect that may inadvertently enhance breeding behaviors. This behavior is also triggered in part by the amount of fruits offered, both fresh and dried. At each annual examination, the same questioning process should be repeated because food habits change as well as what the bird owner provides. Some species, like cockatoos, are able to get owners to feed them only what they want to eat.

It is important to determine how much of each food group is being consumed. The food groups that are used with companion psittacines include fruits, vegetables, protein sources, cereals, and grains including seeds and nuts. In addition, it should be determined whether and how much balanced nutritional food is consumed. Balanced foods include extruded or pelleted diets or Lafeber Nutri-Berries and/or Avi-Cakes (Lafeber Company, Cornell, IL). Seed mixes with pellets added to balance the ration

Table 2
Nutrient profile recommendations for psittacine and passerine birds

Nutrient		General Psittacine Profile		General Passerine Profile	
		Minimum Level	Maximum Level	Minimum Level	Maximum Level
	Gross energy (kcal/kg)	3200	4200	3500	4500
	Total protein (%)	12	—	14	—
Amino acids	Linoleic acid (%)	1	—	1	—
	Lysine (%)	0.65	—	0.75	—
	Methionine (%)	0.30	—	0.35	—
	Methionine plus cysteine (%)	0.50	—	0.58	—
	Arginine (%)	0.65	—	0.75	—
	Threonine (%)	0.40	—	0.46	—
Vitamins, fat soluble	Vitamin A activity (total) (IU/kg)	8000	—	8000	—
	Vitamin D_3 (ICU/kg)	500	2000	1000	2500
	Vitamin E (ppm)	50	—	50	—
	Vitamin K (ppm)	1.0	—	1.0	—
Vitamins, water soluble	Thiamine (ppm)	4.0	—	4.0	—
	Riboflavin (ppm)	6.0	—	6.0	—
	Niacin (ppm)	50.0	—	50.0	—
	Pyridoxine (ppm)	20.0	—	20.0	—
	Pantothenic acid (ppm)	20.0	—	20.0	—
	Biotin (ppm)	0.25	—	0.25	—
	Folic acid (ppm)	1.50	—	1.50	—
	Vitamin B_{12} (ppm)	0.01	—	0.01	—
	Choline (ppm)	1500	—	1500	—
Minerals	Calcium (%)	0.30	1.20	0.50	1.20
	Phosphorus, total (%)	0.30	—	0.50	—
	Calcium/total phosphorus	1:1	2:1	1:1	2:1
	Potassium (%)	0.40	—	0.40	—
	Sodium (%)	0.12	—	0.12	—
	Chlorine (%)	0.12	—	0.12	—
	Magnesium (ppm)	600	—	600	—
Trace minerals	Manganese (ppm)	65.0	—	65.0	—
	Iron (ppm)	80.0	—	80.0	—
	Zinc (ppm)	50.0	—	50.0	—
	Copper (ppm)	8.0	—	8.0	—
	Iodine (ppm)	0.40	—	0.40	—
	Selenium (ppm)	0.10	—	0.10	—

From Hawley SB. Year-end report of the nutrition and management committee, AAV Annual Meeting. Tampa, August 27, 1996; and *Reprinted from* Hawley B, Ritzman T, Edline TM. Avian nutrition. In: Olsen GH, Orosz SE, editors. Manual of avian nutrition. St Louis (MO): Mosby; 2000. p. 378–9.

are not, in fact, balanced, because birds rarely eat the few pellets that are added. This process of nutritional history taking is done to determine whether the overall diet is balanced. Not all companion birds exclusively eat pellets. Only providing a pelleted or extruded diet is not practical or the way to approach health, particularly in highly intelligent avian species. Owners want to provide other foods and these need to be factored in to determine whether the overall diet is nutritionally balanced. To do that, the veterinarian should determine whether there is sufficient protein, vitamins, and minerals.

From the history, it is important to determine whether the fat-soluble vitamins (vitamins A, D_3, E, and K) are adequate in the diet consumed. In addition, from the nutritional history, it is important to assess whether the calcium levels are appropriate, along with phosphorus. It is more difficult to determine whether the amino acids are balanced.

From a potential training perspective, the avian patient's favorite food item(s) should be listed as well. As a greater understanding develops that natural behaviors are linked to foraging, part of the history should document the use and the extent of foraging for the bird to meet its daily dietary requirement. The veterinarian should then be able to discuss with the client ways to help the bird forage for food. When I try to explain that the goal is to no longer use food bowls or cups but to provide the bird's daily nutritional requirement through foraging, they often understand what we are trying to accomplish. Part of the nutritional information provided in the examination room may need to include how to get that patient to forage, because birds vary both in foraging experience and preferences. Further, different foraging methods suit different species. For example, cockatoos are able to use complex foraging opportunities, particularly with plastic puzzles linked to food, whereas cockatiels are not.

How water is provided and how often it is changed should be recorded as well. Another factor to determine is what the expectations of the owner are in their relationship with the bird, which helps to determine success in feed conversion, level of foraging, and level of training for behavior modification.

However, most companion birds are fed seed-only diets and most owners do not seek a veterinarian to receive nutritional advice. Some companion birds are offered pellets along with seed. Others use a seed diet with a few pellets mixed in and those can be labeled as balanced. However, when asked, owners often admit that the bird never eats the pellets in those mixtures. It is therefore important to determine the amount of each food item consumed.

It is important to explain in a nonconfrontational way that seed-only diets are deficient in fat-soluble vitamins and major minerals (Ca, PO_4, Na, Mn, Zn, Fe, I, Se), that they are often high in fats, and that the amino acids are unbalanced. Seed-only diets have been found to be deficient in the amino acids lysine, methionine, riboflavin, pantothenic acid, niacin, and choline.[4] The importance of feeding these fat-soluble vitamins also needs to be explained or shown. We have a few clinic birds on balanced diets in our veterinary hospital and taking clients alongside their cages and showing them the differences in the quality of the feathering, sheen, and skin, for example, between their birds and the birds on a balanced diet is often impressive enough to motivate change. Just telling owners that seed-only diets are deficient in various vitamins and minerals is not enough. How these food components affect the health of their bird needs to be explained as well. The following information provides a basis for that discussion. It will also help to determine whether the bird is closer or further from a balanced diet.

VITAMINS
Vitamin A

Vitamin A is the vitamin that is most likely to be deficient in the diets of both captive and wild birds because the amount consumed in foodstuffs can be variable. Vitamin A represents all noncarotenoid derivatives that have a biological activity similar to all transretinols. Most appear as retinol and retinol esters that are absorbed from the gastrointestinal tract and transported by portomicrons for storage in the liver.[1]

There are 2 basic functions of vitamin A in cells: the hormonelike regulatory actions of retinoic acid and the photoreceptor actions of retinal. The hormonelike action involves binding to nuclear and cytoplasmic receptors to induce the regulation of cellular replication, differentiation, and preprogrammed cell death. For example, without adequate levels of vitamin A, the basal cells of the respiratory and gastrointestinal tracts differentiate into a keratinized squamous epithelium instead of their normal morphology.[1]

The exact requirement of vitamin A is unknown in psittacine birds. Feeding trials in female cockatiels suggest that the range may be between 2000 and 10,000 IU/kg in this species because there were no clinical signs that the birds experienced signs of a deficiency or toxicity. Cockatiels could be maintained for 8 months with no dietary vitamin A, although they showed signs of immune incompetence, suggesting that the levels required in these species is probably low.[1]

However, less grain-dependent species may have greater requirements than the low levels required by cockatiels. Psittacine birds deficient in vitamin A have several problems, including showing signs of keratinization of their mucous membranes, anorexia, poor conditioning, and increased susceptibility to infection. Parrots also show metaplasia of the salivary glands, including their excretory ducts and glandular epithelium. The choanal papillae are often blunted and the slit is widened with chronic deficiency. Vocalizations in cockatiels may be affected by vitamin A status, because cockatiels fed a diet high in vitamin A (100,000 IU vitamin A/kg diet) had increased numbers of vocalizations compared with birds fed 2000 IU/kg. Cockatiels fed a diet entirely deficient in vitamin A had reduced peak amplitude and total power of vocalization.[1]

Vitamin A deficiency impairs the function of the rods in the eyes and causes night blindness in birds. However, this can be reversible with feeding adequate levels of vitamin A in just a few days if caught early.[5] Severe deficiencies result in keratinization of the conjunctiva with inadequate lubrication of the cornea, which creates abrasions and possible loss of sight.

A Gram stain of the choanal cells provides a quick assessment of vitamin A/beta carotenoid levels in the avian patient. When levels are adequate the choanal cells on a Gram stain are lightly eosinophilic to lightly basophilic. When the vitamin A levels deviate significantly from normal they appear as immature cells that are moderately to highly basophilic. Chronic vitamin A deficiency leads to hyperkeratotic cells with sharp borders and that are moderately to highly eosinophilic.

Carotenoids in the diet (**Fig. 1**) serve as vitamin A precursors in chickens and it is assumed that psittacines also use them in a similar manner. Beta carotene and other carotenoids can be degraded enzymatically in the intestinal epithelium to form retinal, one form of vitamin A, which can then be converted to other forms such as retinol and retinoic acid. The role of dietary carotenoids for pigmentation of feathers is not known, because even cockatiels on vitamin A–free diets maintained their pigmentation. In

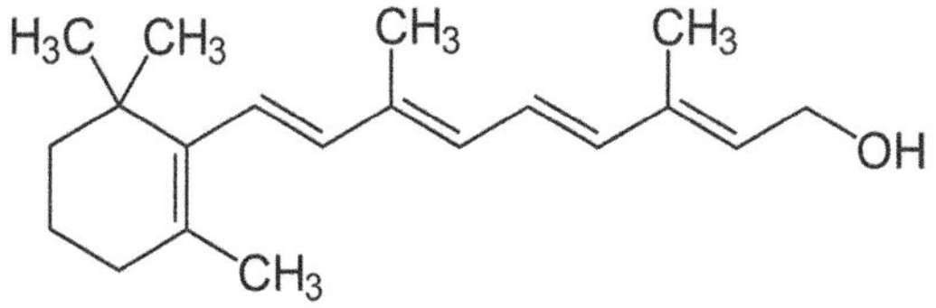

Fig. 1. Retinol, a form of vitamin A, can be produced from retinal, which results when beta carotenes in the diet are enzymatically degraded.

contrast, Canaries depend on carotenoids in their diets to enhance the yellow/orange in their feathering.

Dietary sources of vitamin A for raptors include the liver and fat of vertebrate prey.[6] Wild birds often have fluctuating stores of vitamin A in their livers because ducks consuming barley and/or wheat become deficient in vitamin A. Of the domestic grains, corn is a rich source of beta carotenes.[5] Sources for companion birds vary from orange, red, and green vegetables to the yolk of the cooked egg. Parsley, pumpkin, yellow squashes, and sweet potato are high in beta carotenes. Egg yolk is the only source of true retinyl esters of vitamin A found in foods from the kitchen.[5]

Toxicity from vitamin A leads to symptoms that are similar to those observed with a deficiency. Dietary history helps to determine the levels of vitamin A and may help distinguish one symptom from another on Gram stains and by clinical observations. High levels of retinoic acid disrupt the differentiation of mucous epithelial cells, resulting in hyperplasia. Hyperplasia can result in the development of necrotic discharges and pustules in the oropharynx, nares, and the area around the globes. T-lymphocyte function declines when retinoic acid levels are high. Retinal is more toxic than retinol because it is easily converted to retinoic acid. The conversion of the carotenoids to vitamin A is regulated in general to the needs of the body. For this reason, consumption of beta carotenoids is a safer alternative than feeding vitamin A directly.[5] Consumption of large amounts of beta carotenes usually does not cause toxicity.

Vitamin D

Vitamin D activity (**Fig. 2**) is found in a group of related sterols including cholecalciferol (vitamin D_3), ergosterol (vitamin D_2), and other metabolites. Birds are able to synthesize cholecalciferol in their skin from cholesterol but require an adequate amount of sunlight to do so. Because most companion birds do not have sufficient ultraviolet exposure for endogenous conversion, they need to have a dietary source of vitamin D. In general, birds are not able to convert D_2, the form available for cats and dogs, into vitamin D_3 for use in metabolism. Instead this form of vitamin D is excreted in the bile.[5]

Vitamin D_3 has hormonal actions because it regulates calcium and phosphorus metabolism, including bone mineralization and eggshell formation. Vitamin D–deficient hens lay eggs with thin shells and develop osteomalacia with pathologic fractures. Vitamin D is taken up by the embryo and converted in the developing kidney to the active form, vitamin D_3. This active hormone causes the uptake of calcium from the yolk sac membranes in the developing embryo and during the later stages it mediates the uptake from the shell via the chorioallantoic membrane.[5]

Birds do not have a requirement for vitamin D_3 if they receive adequate sunlight. However, the established requirement in chickens (200 mg/kg diet) to turkeys

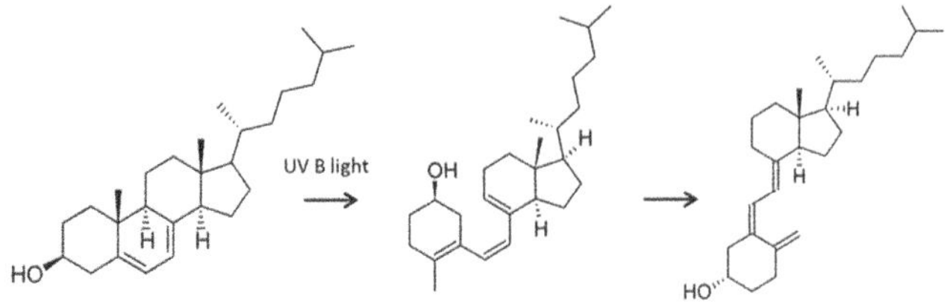

7-Dehydrocholesterol   Previtamin D_3 Cholecalciferol

Fig. 2. Conversion of 7-dehydrocholesterol to cholecalciferol (vitamin D_3) in the skin of birds with the aid of ultraviolet light.

(1100 mg/kg diet)[2] is based on the assumption that no exogenous synthesis occurs. In addition, as calcium levels decrease, phosphorus levels in the diet increase, or the Ca/PO_4 ratio is either too high or too low, the dietary requirement of vitamin D_3 increases. However, birds are able to use 25(OH)2D_3 and/or 1,25(OH)2D_3 as a dietary source for preventing bone diseases or treating these problems.

Vitamin D toxicity is associated with increased mobilization of calcium with soft tissue mineralization including joints, kidneys, myocardium, blood vessels, and the pancreas. In the kidney, tubule calcification can result in a fatal buildup of excretory products.[5] Unpublished data suggest that increased levels of vitamin D in hand-feeding diets in psittacines can result in renal failure (Phalen D, unpublished data, 2003). Most commonly in companion birds, high levels of vitamin D_3 have come from pelleted or extruded diets in which the levels were too high. Vitamin D toxicity seems to vary considerably by species; a vitamin D toxicity was induced in several species of macaw parrots at levels considerably lower than the levels tolerated by most other species (1,000,000 IU vitamin D_3/kg dry matter).[5]

Vitamin E

Vitamin E consists of 2 groups of compounds with antioxidant activity, the alpha-tocopherols (**Fig. 3**) and the gamma-tocotrienols. The most biologically active form of vitamin E is the D-tocopherol, which is used as the dietary standard. In birds, it seems that only the alpha-tocopherols are incorporated into tissues.[5] Vitamin E is transported by plasma lipoproteins and incorporated into the lipid bilayer of the cell's membranes. It acts to stabilize these membranes and to quench reactions of oxygen intermediates and polyunsaturated fatty acids. These alpha-tocopherols can compete for free radicals faster than polyunsaturated fatty acids. They can also work in concert with several enzymes, including superoxide dismutase, glutathione peroxidase, and catalase, to protect cell membranes. These enzymes require some of the trace minerals, including zinc, manganese, selenium, and iron, as cofactors for proper function. When deficient, the absolute requirement of vitamin E increases, showing that many of the nutrients are linked.

Vitamin E has other physiologic effects primarily through modulation of eicosanoid metabolism. Conversion of arachidonic acid into prostaglandins and thromboxanes can be modulated by vitamin E levels, which results in alteration of the immune responses to a challenge.

The levels of vitamin E required in the diet vary, depending on several factors, including the levels of polyunsaturated fatty acids, levels of vitamin A and/or beta carotene, the presence and quantity of other dietary antioxidants, rancidity of the fats in the diet, and the content of selenium. A selenium deficiency results in an impairment of the glutathione peroxidase antioxidant system, increasing the need for vitamin E.

Deficiencies of vitamin E result in several symptoms that relate to cell membrane dysfunctions. These commonly observed symptoms include encephalomalacia, exudative diathesis, muscular dystrophy, myopathy of the ventriculus, and increased

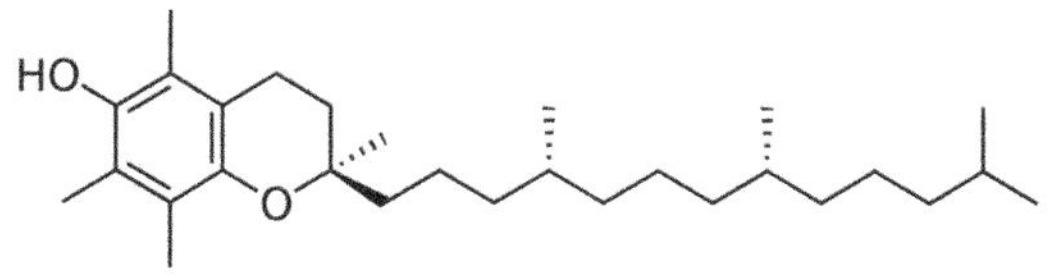

Fig. 3. Alpha tocopherol, a form of vitamin E. Other forms exist and vary in the number and position of methyl groups.

fragility of red blood cells. Encephalomalacia in chicks results in crazy chick disease, characterized by torticollis, crying out, and excessive wing flapping while maintaining abnormal postures. Higher than normal levels of vitamin E can result in the symptoms associated with deficiencies of the other fat-soluble vitamins. The bioactivity of vitamin E is drastically reduced during processing because of heat and moisture, along with increased levels of unsaturated fatty acids and trace minerals.[5] Poultry have a low level of toxicity to vitamin E and levels greater than 100 times the requirement are well tolerated.

Vitamin E is synthesized only by plants and alpha-tocopherols are mainly found in leaves of plants; gamma tocopherols are found more commonly in grains and vegetable oils but the most active form of vitamin E in birds is alpha-tocopherol. Foods high in vitamin E include green leafy vegetables, egg yolks, palm nuts, and canola oil.

Vitamin K

Vitamin K is a group of compounds that are related to menadione (2-methyl-1,4 naphthoquinone of vitamin K_3) that show antihemorrhagic activity. Menadione is a common synthetic form of vitamin K. Vitamin K functions as a cofactor of a hepatic microsomal carboxylase that catalyzes the posttranslational carboxylation of specific glutamate residues. This carboxylation is important for the function of at least 12 proteins that include osteocalcin; clotting factors VII, IX, and X; and prothrombin. Vitamin K turns over rapidly in tissues compared with other fat-soluble vitamins and is not stored for periods of time in the liver.

The low concentration of this enzyme needed in the body results in a low requirement. Even though its requirement is low, vitamin K is important for the clotting mechanism. Because this vitamin is excreted in the feces, coprophagy can help to provide the daily requirement. Vitamin K requirements increase with infection and with the presence of vitamin K antagonists. These antagonists can include dicumarols produced by molds from grains and antibiotics administered during long-term regimens that deplete normal intestinal microflora. Domestic ducks are particularly sensitive to vitamin K depletion from antibiotic therapy. Psittacines with liver failure and consuming seed-only diets have had uncontrolled hemorrhage, usually from a broken blood feather in a practice setting.

Vitamin K is usually supplemented with a water-soluble form of menadione to reduce possible toxicity but chickens are tolerant of more than 1000 times the normal requirement. Leaves of plants are rich sources of vitamin K, whereas fruits and seeds are poor, along with soybean meal.[5]

OMEGA FATTY ACIDS

The polyunsaturated fatty acids (PUFAs) of the n-6 and n-3 (**Fig. 4**) series affect immunity and its response, and cardiovascular and nervous system health, and also improve renal function and reduce arthritis. The PUFAs are thought to affect the immune function in 3 basic ways: altering eicosanoid synthesis, changing cell membranes that affect membrane-associated protein and receptor functions, and changing fatty acid pools that affect cytokine production. In general, PUFAs of the omega 3 series tend to produce fewer inflammatory cytokines. The n-6 PUFA arachidonic acid is the precursor for prostaglandins, leukotrienes, and other related compounds that produce proinflammatory cytokines. Several studies have examined the antiinflammatory role of the n-3 PUFA on fish oils, eicosapentaenoic acid, and docosahexaenoic acid in cardiovascular and inflammatory/autoimmune diseases, suggesting that they have a beneficial effect.[7]

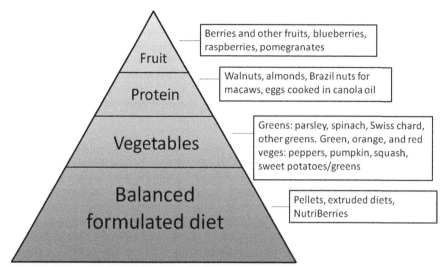

Fig. 4. Formulated diets should form the base of the avian companion bird's diet, followed by smaller fractions of vegetables, nuts and other protein sources, and a small serving of fruit (true berries preferred).

In the history, it is important to establish whether the avian patient is receiving balanced PUFAs, because most birds are not. Seeds and grains, in general, are too high in the n-6/n-3 PUFA ratio, which contributes to the unkempt appearance of the feathers, reduction of sheen, and possible feather chewing from itchiness. These physical manifestations of an improper ratio can be used to help clients understand the need to steer their bird from a seed-only diet toward balanced nutrition. Some formulated diet manufacturers (eg, Lafeber Company) balance the PUFAs, and other food manufacturers are following suit as well. Supplementation with balanced PUFA oils may help, along with eggs cooked in canola oil, walnuts, and flax seeds (Klasing KC, personal communication, 2006).

MINERALS

The mineral required in the largest quantity is calcium. It is necessary for bone mineralization and eggshell calcification, and its ionic form is required for nerve conduction and for myofibril contraction. The calcium requirement(s) for psittacine species have not been determined but the maintenance requirement for chickens is 0.1% of the diet. Many of the seeds consumed by companion birds are less than 0.03% of the diet, suggesting that the requirement is larger than 0.05%. African gray parrots are particularly prone to hypocalcemic seizures. The pathophysiology is unknown but the condition may result from an inability to mobilize bone acutely or from other causes unrelated to nutrition. This problem seems less apparent clinically when birds eat at least half of their diet as pellets because vitamin D_3 is provided. African grays are one species that has a uropygial gland and, consequently, they may have a higher requirement or sensitivity for cholecalciferol when not exposed to sunlight. Sunlight is needed to convert the inactive form of vitamin D to the active form, or it needs to be supplied on a regular basis.

The requirement for growing psittacine chicks is unknown, but they are expected to require a similar calcium/phosphorous ratio (between 1.4:1 and 4:1), assuming the vitamin D levels are adequate. The calcium requirement for altricial species of birds is less than that of precocial species because the number and size per egg is greater in the latter birds. The calcium requirement in egg-laying chicken hens is 3.3% of the diet, whereas budgerigars and cockatiels require as little as 0.85% and 0.35%, respectively, for normal calcification.[8,9] Calcium deficiency occurs when there is too little calcium or the active form of vitamin D or too much phosphorus in the diet. The lack of calcium and the active form of vitamin D in all-seed diets is the underlying problem with egg binding in cockatiels.

PROTEIN AND AMINO ACIDS

The essential amino acids for birds are arginine, isoleucine, leucine, lysine, methionine, phenylalanine, valine, tryptophan, and threonine. Research with chickens suggests that glycine, histidine, and proline are also considered essential because their rates of synthesis are less than their metabolic needs. Research in budgerigars also suggests that, unlike chickens, they cannot synthesize enough glycine and that it is an essential amino acid for them as well. One common problem is obesity in budgerigars and Amazons on all-seed diets. It is presumed that the birds will continue to consume these diets seeking to meet their amino acid requirements. However, because these diets are deficient in some of the amino acids, they are unable to meet those needs and, in the process, get fat.

Protein levels consumed must meet the nitrogen requirements for that species in its housing condition and life stage. Growing chicks require greater amounts of protein, especially hatchlings. Hens laying large clutches of eggs also require larger amounts of protein than those at maintenance. Birds within a dietary strategy (eg, granivorous birds) that have an increased body size also have higher protein requirements than smaller species.

Feathers compose the largest portion of the protein mass of birds. In budgerigars, they represent 5.7% of the protein mass, which is 28% of the total body protein. Molt results in increased protein needs and these needs differ from those of the general body. Feathers are enriched with cysteine and many of the nonessential amino acids. These amino acids are incorporated into the feather during its formation on a continual basis, whereas uptake from the gastrointestinal tract occurs only after consumption of a meal, requiring that they be manufactured from tissue protein sources. Molt is also expensive energetically because the bird loses insulation during that period, consequently requiring increased energy. There are also increased expenditures to acquire more protein to synthesize feather proteins.

Protein digestibility is assumed to be similar in the granivorous psittacines, compared with chickens. This assumption is based on the assimilation efficiencies of complete diets, which are similar in psittacines and chickens.[1] The quality of the protein in the diet reflects the digestibility of the components and the amino acid balance. Rate-limiting amino acids require that more food be consumed to meet that need, which may lead to obesity. If more food is not consumed, a clinically observed deficiency may result. For example, methionine deficiency during chick growth results in dark stress bars on feathers.[10]

High-protein diets have been assumed to lead to gout in birds, but this supposition has not been supported by research. Adult male cockatiels, when fed diets with up to 70% crude protein for 11 months, maintained their body weight and general body condition without evidence of renal dysfunction. There was evidence of liver damage because birds developed sinusoidal and periportal lipogranulomas at the 70% level, but not at the 20% or 35% levels. It seems that sudden changes to high-protein diets might lead to hyperuricacidemia with possible nephritis or gout.[1] However, there is no research at present that indicates that this hypothesis is valid. However, sudden changes are not recommended.

FORMULATED DIETS

Formulated balanced diets for psittacines include (1) pellets; (2) extruded foods, which are often termed pellets; and (3) whole grains and/or seeds with pelleted material packed between the components to balance the product, such as Nutri-Berries and Avi-Cakes (Lafeber Company).

From a label perspective, the balance is not stated but implied because most of these diets represent variations of a balanced diet for galliforms or a diet prepared according to the AAV panel recommendations (see **Table 1**). There are few nutritional studies on maintenance requirements for this large group of psittacine species with diverse ecological niches, and this limitation is compounded by the other need to better understand the nutritional requirements of life stages of a particular species.

True pellets are made by grinding a variety of grains based on the manufacturer's recommendations and, to that ground mix, vitamins and minerals are added to make the final product balanced. Grinding reduces particle size to make it easier to produce a homogeneous mixture. This process is used so that the bird is unable to pick out and eat the components of the food that it likes. By grinding and mixing the food, it ensures that the bird receives this balanced diet. Once ground, the mix is commonly put through a hammer mill to ensure appropriate particle size. Liquids may then be added and the ground mix pelleted. Pelleting uses a dry or steam process under heat (often at 70–80°C [158–176°F]) whereby the mix is heated and forced through holes in a die using a roller. As it emerges as cylindrical particles of a constant diameter, a turning knife cuts the pellets as preset lengths.[11]

Most of the so-called pellets that are available today are really extruded diets. These diets are made by mixing ground grains with the vitamin and mineral components that balance the final formula. This mix is then forced through an extruder, which may involve a dry process or a steam process using an injection technique. The mix is then forced under pressure and temperature (90–180°C [194–356°F]) through the extruder with a dwell time from 30 seconds to several minutes. Moisture added as steam may be between 0% and 20%. The holes in the plate of the extruder determine the shape of the food pieces. The pressure helps maintain the water in a liquid state. The rapid expansion on leaving the extruder causes instantaneous evaporation of intracellular water, rupturing the plant cells. The food produced is partially hydrolyzed but the cooking can kill infectious agents if present.[11]

A third strategy is used to formulate Nutri-Berries and Avi-Cakes (Lafeber Company), which use whole grains and seeds that are mixed with a pellet base that balances the product before it is stuck together. It is similar to a pellet except that it is not ground.

There are some seed-based foods to which a pellet is added to balance the seed mixture or a vitamin/mineral mix that is coated on the outside of the seed. However, most birds pick out the seed preferentially from these additions, leaving the remainder behind. As an alternative, seeds may be hull coated. The nutritional result from these formulations may be markedly reduced or produce nutritional imbalances. If the added nutrition is not consumed, the nutritional result may be no better than that of an all-seed diet.

It is important for veterinarians to understand the processes and the issues involved in avian nutrition to advise their clients appropriately to meet the individual needs of their patients. Each bird may have certain factors as well as medical conditions that need to be taken into account when advising owners on how to feed their birds.

FEEDING COMPANION BIRDS IN THE HOME

As indicated, psittacines in the wild do not necessarily select food stuffs that are adequate nutritionally and meet maintenance needs. However, they seem to be able to balance their energy, amino acids, and calcium needs, but not their needs for other requirements. However, birds in captivity do not seem to select appropriately either. A self-selected diet in African gray parrots (*P erithacus*) resulted in a diet that was deficient in a total of 12 dietary components consisting of vitamins, minerals, and amino acids.[4] Owners commonly provide a diet with a large selection of foodstuffs that include birdie breads, chop, and other foods. These owners are well intentioned because they want to provide good nutrition and think that the bird can self-balance its diet. The study by Ullrey and colleagues[4] disputes that supposition. Another problem with the smorgasbord effect is that many psittacines are signaled by this rich diversity of foods and this may contribute to reproductive behaviors. For this reason, it is important to caution clients to provide fewer selections each day, but the choices can vary between days.

Over the past 20 years, the dietary approach suggested by avian veterinarians was to provide a pelleted or extruded mixture that provides all of the required nutrients at greater than the estimated requirements. This approach has greatly improved the health of companion birds compared with an all-seed diet. However, there is reluctance by owners to use pelleted diets. One problem expressed by clients is that they are unable to convert their birds to a pelleted or extruded diet. There is also a concern about the lack of variety for species that often have a huge selection of food items in the wild; these diets offer no opportunity for birds to display their innate foraging behavior. Another more recent concern is that the foods contain harmful components for the birds and so it is better to provide chop and other foods.

The addition of vegetables and fruits to a diet of pellets for variety and for enrichment suggests that nutrient dilution may occur. In theory, that requires that the diet be reformulated to increase the nonenergy portion of the diet to reduce this problem. However, this problem becomes more of an issue when the bird is eating a smaller portion of the diet as a balanced diet (<50%) than table foods offered. The reason that this may not be observed commonly is that most domestic fruits and vegetables are predominately water. A serving of fruit such as a fresh berry each day is preferred to dried fruits because dried fruits concentrate sugars; fruits high in simple sugars include the common grape and banana (Klasing KC, personal communication, 2006). Overall, formulated diets should form the base of the avian companion bird's diet, followed by smaller fractions of vegetables, nuts, and other protein sources, and a small serving of fruit (true berries preferred) (**Fig. 5**).

CONVERSION OF SMALL BIRDS SUCH AS BUDGERIGARS, COCKATIELS, LOVEBIRDS, AND CONURES

Cockatiels and budgerigars are ground-feeding granivores in their native habitats. They are able to balance their diets because of the large numbers of seeds that they eat (more than 60 types).[1] However, the number and the types of the seeds offered in people's homes are significantly less and are not similar, so the birds need a balanced diet to maintain health. To stimulate their interest, try sprinkling a

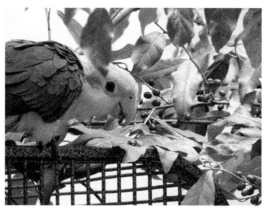

Fig. 5. Home environments can be enriched to provide foraging opportunities. In this case, a white-bellied caique consumes berries from an autumn olive shrub.

few small pellets on the table along with some crumbled Nutri-Berries. To get them interested, we suggest that the client acts enthusiastically as the bird starts pecking at the scattered foods. Clients are counseled to use a forefinger and thumb to pick these pieces up. That excitement translates into curiosity for these new foods and helps the avian patient to accept them.

Once the birds start pecking and eating these balanced foods, these new food items can be mixed into the food bowl with their seed. Crumbled Nutri-Berries or Avi-Cakes may also be used because they look like the seeds that are being substituted. Add increasing amounts of the balanced diet slowly, so that over time the seed is replaced with these new balanced foods. Clients may also wedge an Avi-Cake into the bars of the cage or tie it with some ribbon. Many of the birds like the texture of the Avi-Cakes and the Avi-Cakes can be used for enrichment as well.

CONVERSION OF LARGE BIRDS SUCH AS AFRICAN GRAYS, AMAZON PARROTS, COCKATOOS, AND MACAWS

Getting these birds to accept new foods presents a different type of challenge. In general, they are not ground feeders so the technique described earlier for small birds often does not work. However, the curiosity factor is important as well as the visual impact of the owner seeming to eat this new and interesting food. Birds are highly visual and typically like drama, so the two combined stimulate their interest in trying this new thing. Instruct the owner to pick up the food with great drama and show interest in relishing these morsels. Offer the food for several seconds and, if the bird does not show any interest, have the owner be very dramatic about coveting this special food. Then present the food again. It may take several sessions at home to get the bird to try these new balanced foods.

Have the owner eat with the bird; giving some of these foods while eating helps the birds to understand that these items are foods to eat. Fresh vegetables; hard scrambled eggs in canola oil; cooked meat and fish; and some of the true berries, mango, and nuts (particularly walnuts) are great additions. Peanuts should be avoided because of the potential for aflatoxins. Instruct the owner to keep the table foods to no more than 25% to 35% of the diet, with the balanced foods making up the remainder.

ENRICHMENT AND FORAGING

Enrichment involves providing an environment that allows the client's bird to express its natural behaviors in a captive or caged condition. Natural behaviors generally include social interaction, foraging, and feather care. Foraging often includes flying from place to place for the gathering of food. As more is learned about ways to provide foraging opportunities, changes will emerge in how companion birds are fed in captivity. Snyder and colleagues[12] documented that Puerto Rican Amazon parrots (*Amazona vittata*) spend approximately 4 to 6 hours per day foraging and that they routinely travel several miles between sites. In contrast, companion birds (orange-winged Amazons [*Amazona amazonica*]) in human homes spend approximately 30 to 72 minutes per day eating a pelleted diet[13] without traveling or manipulating food items, and not attempting to balance their own diets.[14] These highly social and intelligent birds need a job to do each day because in the wild they are foraging.

Linking foraging foods with objects enhances the birds' captive behaviors and brain stimulation. To satisfy their natural foraging behavioral repertoire, birds in home environments need to learn to forage in their cages to acquire their food.

Studies indicate that linking a food item with an object or toy that allows the expression of their natural behaviors results in more successful use of that toy.[14] In contrast, the frequency of use of toys not linked to a food item often diminishes over time as the bird loses interest. Therefore, it is important to provide daily enrichment opportunities that involve chewing and manipulating a food item.

One technique to show clients is to wrap a food item that the bird likes to eat in a small paper kitchen cup. Show the bird the cup and the food item in a dramatic manner and then wrap it in front of it. Then hand it to the bird. Some birds will at least take it from the veterinarian in the examination room. Others are not comfortable, so they can take the item home to try there. Start with a clear plan on foraging steps and have the owner call at an appointed time.

What to expect from a cockatoo is different from what to expect from an Amazon. Cockatoos are adept at and enjoy unscrewing large wing nuts and taking things apart. They often like plastic ropes with plastic beads tied into them to take apart. They are the engineers of the psittacine world. Amazons and macaws just chew their way through things instead. African grays like color and sound. Conures like to chew, particularly on paper, and are interested in textures. The type of foraging toy and its size therefore need to suit the species. Guiding clients is important so that they

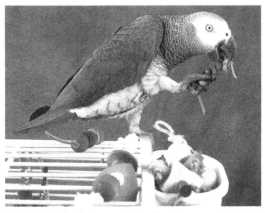

Fig. 6. This African gray is manipulating wooden beads strung on a leather strap.

become more attuned to their birds and interact with them in a positive way. That process helps to strengthen the human–companion bird bond and helps to maintain a good relationship (**Fig. 6**).

ACKNOWLEDGMENTS

The information provided presents principles of nutrition that I have gained by working with Dr Kirk Klasing, to whom I am indebted. I have translated the knowledge gained to a clinical setting to help my avian patients lead better lives. This work was started by inspiration from Dr T.J. Lafeber when I was first in practice and later when he discussed ideas while I was a faculty member at The University of Tennessee. His son, Dr Ted Lafeber, has continued to push me along in my understanding of nutrition. All have been inspirational, along with my feathered patients.

REFERENCES

1. Koutsos EA, Matson KD, Klasing KC. Nutrition of birds in the order Psittaciformes: a review. J Avian Med Surg 2001;15:257–75.
2. National Research Council. Nutrient requirements of poultry. Washington, DC: National Academy Press; 1994.
3. Hawley B, Ritzman T, Edling TM. Avian nutrition. In: Olsen GH, Orosz SE, editors. Manual of avian medicine. St Louis (MO): Mosby; 2000. p. 369–90.
4. Ullrey DE, Allen ME, Baer DJ. Formulated diets versus seed mixtures for psittacines. J Nutr 1991;121:S193–205.
5. Klasing KC. Vitamins. In: Klasing KC, editor. Comparative avian nutrition. New York: CABI Publishing; 1998. p. 277–329.
6. Dierenfeld ES, Sandfort CE, Satterfield WC. Influence of diet on plasma vitamin E in captive peregrine falcons. J Wildl Manage 1989;53:160–4.
7. Anderson M, Fritsche KL. (n-3) Fatty acids and infectious disease resistance. J Nutr 2002;132:3566–76.
8. Earle KE, Clarke NR. The nutrition of the budgerigar (*Melopsittacus undulatus*). J Nutr 1991;121:186S–92S.
9. Roudybush T. Nutrition. In: Rosskopf W, Woerpel R, editors. Diseases of cage and aviary birds. Baltimore (MD): Williams & Wilkins; 1996. p. 218–34.
10. MacWhirter P. Malnutrition. In: Ritchie BW, Harrison GJ, Harrison LR, editors. Avian medicine: principles and application. Lake Worth (FL): Wingers; 1994. p. 842–61.
11. Larbier M, Leclercq B. Processing of diets and nutritional consequences. In: Larbier M, Leclercq B, editors. Nutrition and feeding of poultry. Leicestershire (United Kingdom): Nottingham University Press; 1994. p. 277–90.
12. Snyder NF, Wiley JW, Kepler CB. The parrots of Luquillo: natural history and conservation of the Puerto Rican parrot. Los Angeles (CA): The Western Foundation of Vertebrate Zoology; 1987.
13. Oviatt LA, Millam JR. Breeding behavior of captive orange-winged Amazon parrots. Exotic Bird Rep 1997;9:6–7.
14. Meehan CL, Millam JR, Mench JA. Foraging opportunity and increased physical complexity both prevent and reduce psychogenic feather picking by young Amazon parrots. Appl Anim Behav Sci 2003;80:71–85.

Captive Marsupial Nutrition

Cathy A. Johnson-Delaney, BS, DVM

KEYWORDS

- Nutrition • Marsupial • Macropod • Sugar glider • Opossum • Wallaby

KEY POINTS

- Marsupials have a basal metabolic rate considered two-thirds of eutherian (placental) mammals.
- Diets for captive marsupials are based on what the animals eat in the wild.
- Diets for companion marsupials (sugar gliders, wallabies, Virginia opossums, and short-tailed opossums) have been developed.
- Hand-rearing marsupials requires using different formulations as the joey matures.

INTRODUCTION

Marsupials comprise an interesting group of mammals, which are increasingly being kept as pets (**Table 1**). These animals include the sugar glider (*Petaurus breviceps*), Bennett's wallaby (*Macropus rufogriseus*), tammar wallaby (*Macropus eugenii*), Virgina opossum (*Didelphis virginiana*), and the South American (Brazilian, Gray) short-tailed opossum (*Monodelphis domestica*). Few actual feeding trials have been published, although many anecdotal diets have years of usage with good success. Marsupials have dental and digestive tract adaptations that allow them to use specific niches in their environments. Wild-type diets have been extensively studied in sugar gliders and wallabies.[1–6] Wild-type diets have been observed for the Virginia opossum and the short-tailed opossum.[7–10] Knowing the diet in the wild is instrumental in designing diets used in captivity.

METABOLISM

Discussion of nutrition begins with metabolic rates, which relate energy and food requirements. There are 3 measures of the rate of metabolism: basal metabolic rate (BMR), field metabolic rate (FMR), and maximum sustained metabolic rate (MSMR). These 3 values are not available for all species of marsupials.

Disclosures: None.
Washington Ferret Rescue & Shelter, Box 1034, 11700 Mukilteo Speedway, Suite 201, Mukilteo, WA 98275, USA
E-mail address: cajddvm@hotmail.com

Vet Clin Exot Anim 17 (2014) 415–447
http://dx.doi.org/10.1016/j.cvex.2014.05.006
1094-9194/14/$ – see front matter © 2014 Elsevier Inc. All rights reserved.

Table 1
Summary of data on BMRs of selected marsupials

Species	Body Mass (g)	mLO$_2$ g^{-1}h^{-1a}	kJ kg$^{-0.75}$/d^b	W kg$^{-0.75c}$	%^{d}
		BMR			
Didelphis virginiana	2403	0.380	238	2.71	81
Macropus eugenii	4878	0.283	212	2.42	72
Monodelphis domestica	104	0.608	161	1.83	55
Petaurus breviceps	128	0.692	209	2.38	71

[a] Mass-specific rate of metabolic intensity.
[b] Energetic equivalence of O$_2$ = 21 kJ L^{-1}.
[c] W = 87.72 kJ per day.
[d] Percentage of predicted value equation for eutherians. The "marsupial mean" is 70% of the eutherian.

Data from Hume ID. Metabolic rates and nutrient requirements. In: Marsupial nutrition. Cambridge (United Kingdom): Cambridge Press; 1999. p. 1–34.

- The definition of BMR of an endotherm is the minimum rate of metabolism compatible with endothermy. It is measured by the rate of oxygen consumption (heat production) of a nonreproductive, postabsorptive adult animal at rest (but not asleep) in its thermoneutral zone and not experiencing any physical or psychological stress.[11] In herbivores, a truly postabsorptive state is never fully reached without starving the animal because of the continued nature of digestive function, with constant production of nutrients by the host microbes.[11]
- FMR is the energy cost of free existence. It includes basal metabolism along with the costs of maintenance, thermoregulation, and activity.[11] Measurements of FMR often include other costs associated with growth, fat storage, and reproduction. Reproduction may include additional activity costs involved with defense of breeding territories, courtship, and foraging on behalf of young. FMRs are more variable for a species than BMR. Thus, FMR relates directly to the real world, and BMRs are more widely used for comparisons across species and taxons.[11]
- The MSMR is the highest rate of energy expenditure that an animal can sustain from food intake, without using body energy stores. It has been measured experimentally in small mammals by using combinations of physical activity, cold stress, and lactation.[11]

BMRs

The traditional view is that the BMR of marsupials is about 30% less than that of eutherian (placental) mammals.[10,11] A BMR for the "average marsupial" is considered to be 49 kcal or 204 kJ kg$^{-0.75}$ day^{-1} or 2.33 W kg$^{-0.75}$.[11] Variations in BMR among both marsupials and eutherians are strongly correlated with food habits, activity level, and precision of temperature regulation.[11]

CONSEQUENCES OF A LOW METABOLIC RATE

- One consequence of a low BMR is generally associated with a low body temperature. A low metabolic rate also has several important consequences for animals in terms of nutrient requirements and thus the width of their nutritional niche.[11]
- Other consequences in environmental tolerance and reproductive rate are related not only to an animal's BMR but also to its metabolic scope, which is the extent to which it can increase metabolism above basal to accommodate

high rates of heat loss in cold environments and the energetic costs of a high reproductive potential.
- A low BMR means lower food requirements for maintenance; energy reserves will last longer under adverse conditions.[11]

MAINTENANCE ENERGY REQUIREMENTS OF CAPTIVE MARSUPIALS

In captive wild animals and housed domestic stock, energy additional to basal requirements is needed for feeding, drinking, digestion, absorption, and metabolism of absorbed nutrients, and for postural changes, but little is needed for thermoregulation or other activities. Under these conditions, maintenance energy requirements are often approximately double the BMR. Metabolizable energy is converted to digestible energy using appropriate factors. With few exceptions, maintenance requirements are in the range of 150% to 250% of BMR. There also seems to be a trend for maintenance requirements as a multiple of BMR to decrease with increasing body mass of the species. This trend may reflect both a greater activity increment and greater requirements for thermoregulation in the smaller species, under captive conditions.[11]

FMRs

FMR, or the energy cost of free existence, is routinely measured by the use of doubly labeled water. The oxygen isotope traces both the water and the carbon dioxide in the body, so the difference between washout rates of oxygen and hydrogen is a measure of CO_2 production (metabolic rate). FMR has been measured in 28 species of marsupials (**Table 2** lists 2 species selected for this article).[11]

- FMR is more variable within a species than is the BMR. The main sources of variation can be identified from **Table 2** as being sex, season, and reproductive status.[11] Unlike BMR, a common scaling factor cannot be used to compare FMRs between the 2 therian groups. At a body size range of 240 to 550 g, FMRs of marsupials and eutherians are similar.
- At lower body sizes, FMRs of eutherians are lower. The only dietary comparison that can be made is within the herbivores, for which marsupials and eutherians both scaled to 0.64, which is the slope of the regression equation relating FMR to body mass. Herbivorous eutherians generally had higher FMRs than herbivorous marsupials, regardless of body size.[11]

More useful than FMR for comparative purposes is the ratio of FMR to BMR (calculated by dividing mass-specific FMR by mass-specific BMR). Analysis showed that the ratio decreased with increasing body mass in marsupials, but in eutherians, it increased with increasing body mass. The high ratio of FMR to BMR in small marsupials is consistent with their relatively high maintenance energy requirements in

Table 2
FMR of selected adult marsupials

Species	Cohort	Season	Body Mass (g)	FMR mLCO$_2$ g^{-1} h^{-1}	FMR kJ/d	FMR kJ kg 0.58/d	FMR/BMR
M eugenii	Adult	Summer	4380	0.518	1150	488	1.9
P breviceps	Female	Spring	112	2.563	153	545	3.9
	Male	Spring	135	2.671	192	613	4.1

Data from Hume ID. Metabolic rates and nutrient requirements. In: Marsupial nutrition. Cambridge (United Kingdom): Cambridge Press; 1999. p. 1–34.

captivity. Analysis of marsupial and eutherian FMR:BMRs showed that ratios were similar at large body size (5–8 kg). At small body size (10–20 g), the ratio in marsupials was twice that of eutherians.

METABOLIC SCOPE

The high FMR:BMR ratio of some small marsupial species raises the question of what is the highest rate of metabolism that can be sustained for the long term. Sustained metabolic rates are time-averaged rates of metabolism in free-ranging animals maintaining body mass over periods that are long enough so that metabolism is fueled by food intake rather than by depletion of energy reserves.

- Sustained metabolic rate is equivalent to the FMR of the animal in energy balance. They are less than peak, or burst metabolic rates, which are short term and fueled largely by anaerobic ATP production for energy stores (mainly glycogen).
- Peak metabolic rates are limited to no more than 1 or 2 minutes because of the toxic effects of lactic acid accumulation. During this time, there may be as much as a 100-fold increase in the animal's BMR. In contrast, aerobically fueled sustained metabolic rates are mostly between 2-fold and 5-fold BMR, but can be as low as 1.3 and as high as 7.2 in lactating ground squirrels, as an example.[11]
- These multiples of BMR are termed the animal's *sustained metabolic scope.*[11]

Metabolic rates higher than the MSMR of a species can be maintained over a shorter period in response to cold stress. These rates are fueled aerobically and the animal must maintain a stable body temperature. Such rates are called summit metabolic rates. The difference between summit metabolic rate and the species' BMR is its *metabolic scope.*[11]

- For example, the summit metabolic rate in the South American didelphid *M domestica* was 8 to 9 times BMR.
- Marsupials have lower metabolic rates than eutherians within their thermoneutral zone, but the same metabolic rates as eutherians below thermoneutrality.
- Marsupials and eutherians do not differ in maximal running speeds. These 2 lines of evidence indicate that the numerous consequences of a low BMR do not include restricted thermoregulatory or locomotory responses, and that marsupials have greater *metabolic scopes* than equivalent eutherians.[11]

TORPOR AND HIBERNATION IN MARSUPIALS

The very high rates of metabolism required for maintenance of endothermy in small mammals at low ambient temperatures are not sustainable unless food supply is constant in quality and quantity.

- In the absence of food, the internal energy stores deplete in a relatively short time, while normothermic. These small endotherms can save large amounts of energy by abandoning regulation of body temperature at their normal high levels.
- Heterothermy is particularly common in insectivores, both marsupial and eutherian, because a constant supply of insects is unlikely in the wild, and they cannot ameliorate fluctuations in food availability by caching food as granivores can.

Heterothermy is manifested in 2 related but distinct ways: shallow daily torpor and hibernation, which is a deep and prolonged torpor.

- The 2 states are distinct in terms of average maximum torpor duration (11 hours in daily torpor vs 355 hours in hibernation), mean minimum body temperature (17.4°C [63.3°F] vs 5.8°C [42.4°F]), minimum metabolic rate (0.54 vs 0.04 mL $O_2 g^{-1}$ body mass^{h-1}), and minimum metabolic rate expressed as a percentage of BMR (30% in daily torpor vs 5% in hibernation).[11]
- Daily torpor occurs in South American didelphid opossums (eg, short-tailed opossum) and in Australian dasyurids and small possums from the family Petauridae (sugar glider and Leadbeater's possum).[11] These species are all omnivores that feed on a mixture of plant exudates and arthropods.[11]
- During torpor, body temperature, heart rate, respiration rate, and overall metabolism decrease; the same state may occur during anesthesia if care is not taken to maintain normal awake levels.
- If torpor is induced during anesthesia, it can complicate postoperative recovery (eg, hemorrhage can occur due to the increase in blood pressure that occurs as the body temperature and metabolism return to normal awake levels).[10]

OTHER NUTRIENTS

Relative to energy, water, and protein, there is only limited information on the requirements of marsupials for the micronutrients (vitamins, minerals, and essential fatty acids).

- There is no evidence of unusually high requirements for any micronutrient among marsupials, but there are suggestions that several micronutrients are required by some marsupials in extremely small amounts.[11]

SUMMARY OF METABOLISM POINTS

- The nutritional niche of a species can be defined principally by what it needs in terms of energy and specific nutrients, and how it harvests and extracts those needed nutrients from the food resources available.
- The amount of any particular nutrient required has 2 components: the amount needed for maintenance of the adult animals, and additional amounts needed for growth, reproduction, and free existence.
- Maintenance requirements are often closely related to the species' BMR, but the extent to which requirements are increased beyond maintenance in different physiologic states and by environmental factors depends on many factors.
- Knowledge of the basic biology and ecology of the species is necessary before the likely relative importance of these various physiologic and environmental factors can be appreciated. This knowledge applies particularly to the total energy and thus total food requirements of free-living animals.
- Information from captive animal studies under controlled conditions is vital for describing and understanding mechanism.
- Information from free-living animals in different season, different physiologic states, and different environments is equally vital for interpreting captive results and testing extrapolations from captivity to the wild state.
- Generally, marsupials have lower BMRs than their eutherian counterparts. They have lower maintenance requirements for energy, protein, and water, but at the level of FMRs marsupial-eutherian comparisons are limited by insufficient data.
- Summit metabolic rates of small marsupials are similar to those of small eutherians and thus small marsupials have greater metabolic scopes.

- Greater metabolic scopes in marsupials mean that a low BMR does not translate into limited capacity for thermoregulation or locomotory responses.
- In inadequate environments, a low BMR serves to maximize the life of energy stores.[11]
- Metabolism can be increased in response to high rates of heat loss or reproductive needs, allowing energy reserves to last longer in adverse conditions.[11]

DIETS IN CAPTIVITY

- The success of a diet designed for the captive marsupial depends on knowledge of the natural diet as well as nutrient needs and the digestive physiology.
- Relatively low requirements may also enable marsupials to use poorer quality diets of higher fiber content than analogous eutherians.
- Many marsupial herbivores feed on natural diets that are surprisingly high in fiber. This diet is possible because they have lower requirements for energy and nutrients when compared with their eutherian counterparts.
- There are dental adaptations for resisting or coping with abrasive plants, and a complex digestive tract in which microbial fermentation plays a central role in fiber degradation as well as the ability to recycle urea and degrade and resynthesize protein.
- In captivity, many marsupial herbivores are often fed concentrates that are higher in all facets of nutrition, frequently leading to obesity.[5]
- Improperly designed diets may also contribute to dietary-related disease. Appropriate diets and quantities must be stressed to owners.[10]

SUGAR GLIDER

Sugar gliders are omnivores with several specialized features that the captive diet should aim to use. They possess enlarged lower incisors for chewing into the bark of trees, lengthened fourth digit on the manus that may aid in the extraction of insects from crevices, and an enlarged cecum whose principal function is probably microbial fermentation of the complex associations of polysaccharides in gum (**Fig. 1**).[10,12–14]

- Observations of wild sugar gliders averaged over all seasons show that approximately 40% of foraging time is spent obtaining acacia gum, 30% is spent foraging for arthropods, and 11% is spent obtaining sap from eucalyptus trees (**Fig. 2**). Examination of feces and stomach contents, however, suggests that 49% of arthropods and 48% of gum are actually ingested.
- Manna, pollen, nectar, and honeydew are minor components of the natural diet in all seasons (**Figs. 3–5**).[12]
- **Table 3** has a description of these components. During autumn and winter, plant exudates predominate in their diet, but during spring and summer, they are primarily insectivorous. Moths, beetles, insect larvae, and spiders are preferred over exudates, possibly because of their increased demand for protein associated with breeding.[13]
- BMR measured in 128 g of captive sugar gliders is reported at 209 kJ $kg^{-0.75}$ per day or about 45 kJ per day (11 kcal per day).
- FMR has also been measured in sugar gliders at about 153 kJ per day (approximately 36 kcal) of a 112 g female glider and 192 kJ per day (approximately 46 kcal) for a 135 g male glider, about 4 times BMR.
- Normal captive activity energy requirements might thus be calculated at around 2 times BMR, or between 76.5 kJ and 96 kJ per day^{-1} (18–23 kcal) for animals

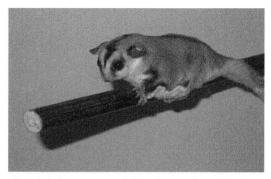

Fig. 1. Sugar glider showing the manus with lengthened fourth digit that aids in extraction of insects from crevices.

averaging approximately 124 g, although some studies suggest higher energy expenditures than this theoretic minimum.[15]

Field energetic studies have demonstrated that wild gliders consume 10.1 to 12.7 g/d of dry food, which provides 182 to 229 kJ/d. This amount is equivalent to approximately 9% of body weight in dry matter per day or about 17% of body weight in fresh food.

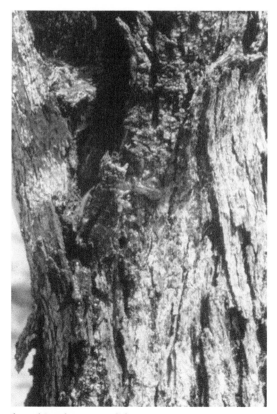

Fig. 2. Sap oozing from bites by sugar gliders.

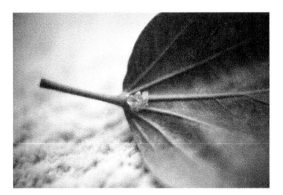

Fig. 3. Manna.

- The captive glider expends less energy in exercise and is generally offered more assimilable foods than the wild glider, so the total energy offered in captivity should be less than or equal to this. Sugar gliders have a BMR similar to that of macropods.[12,13]

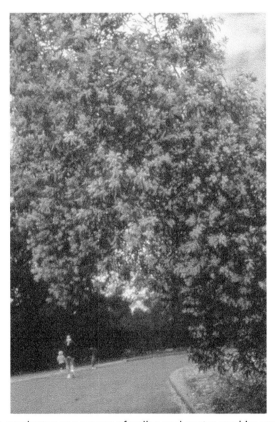

Fig. 4. Flowering eucalyptus as a source of pollen and nectar used by sugar gliders.

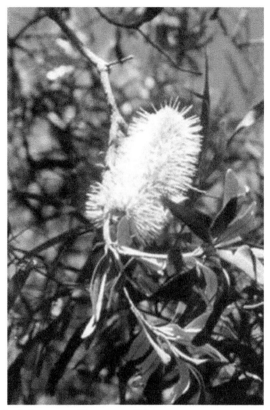

Fig. 5. Flowering Banksia sp. used by sugar gliders.

- The sugar glider has a low maintenance dietary nitrogen requirement of 87 mg kg$^{-0.75}$ per day due to an unusually low loss of metabolic fecal nitrogen (0.7 mg g^{-1} dry matter intake) compared with an average value in herbivorous marsupials of 2.8.[11]
- Endogenous urinary nitrogen (EUN) loss was also low in sugar gliders (25 mg kg$^{-0.75}$ per day) compared with an average value in macropods of 54. EUN is related more closely to the animal's metabolic rate than to any aspect of its protein metabolism.
- The explanation for the sugar gliders' low loss of nitrogen is that part of their endogenous nitrogen is retained by being recycled to the digestive tract. The gums on which it feeds are fermented in the cecum. Their high-energy diet may be expected to result in efficient trapping of recycled nitrogen, resulting in lower urea excretion rates than those of, for example, herbivores feeding on lower-energy plant material.[11,15]

Sugar gliders fed honey-pollen diets containing 1.0%, 3.1%, or 6.5% protein on a dry basis had maintenance nitrogen requirements determined at 87 mg kg$^{-0.75}$ per day, or about 248 mg crude protein for a 100-g animal. Gliders displayed low nitrogen losses in both feces and urine, which may be related to low metabolic rates, overall, or to efficient use of potentially limited resource. Based on these laboratory studies, free-ranging male gliders are likely able to meet minimal protein requirements with diets

Table 3
Definition and composition of dietary components of wild sugar gliders

Component	Definition	Composition
Gum	Exuded on trunks and branches by some species of Acacia to bind sites of damage, particularly those made by insects	Complex associations of polysaccharides (cellulose, starch, and sugars), low in protein (1.3%–3.1%)
Arthropods	Moths, beetles, caterpillars, weevils, and spiders	Vary in composition but contain in the region of 50%–75% protein, and 5%–20% fat on a dry weight basis
Sap	Liquid obtained by biting through the bark of some eucalyptus trees into the phloem	1.4% or less protein, predominantly carbohydrate, of which 70%–85% is sucrose
Manna	Sugary exudates produced at sites of insect damage on the leaves and branches of certain eucalyptus and angophoras	Composition of sugars slightly changed from phloem sap by the action of insects' salivary enzymes
Honeydew	Sap-sucking insects ingest large quantities of sap to obtain sufficient protein and then excrete surplus carbohydrates as honeydew	About 79% monosaccharides and oligosaccharides and 9% polysaccharides
Nectar	Produced in usable quantities by larger eucalyptus flowers (>5 mm in diameter)	Many simple sugars

Data from Booth RJ. General husbandry and medical care of sugar gliders. In: Bonagura JD, editor. Kirk's current veterinary therapy XIII. Philadelphia: WB Saunders; 2000. p. 1157–63.

comprising exudates alone, but female gliders must supplement with pollen or arthropods to meet demands of reproduction.[11]

A recent feeding trial comparing 3 diets in young, growing male gliders averaging 96 g found animals consumed 100.1 kJ to 147 kJ (24–35 kcal) per day.[15] Sugar gliders do not hibernate but can display shallow daily torpor periods, with a drop in body temperature from about 35°C (95°F), to 11°C (51.8°F), to 28°C (82.4°F) for several hours, accompanied by decreases in metabolic rate to 10% to 60% of basal metabolism, mainly in response to food restriction.[15]

The suitability of the captive diet can be judged by monitoring body weight, body condition, coat condition, and fecal consistency.

- Despite the current detailed knowledge and the fact that gliders have been kept as pets for several years, many still present for veterinary care with problems related to improper feeding, including malnutrition, osteodystrophy, and dental disease.[15,16]
- Obesity is a common problem in captivity. Captive animals are often fed an excess quantity of food, excess simple sugars, and excess fat, combined with insufficient exercise.
- The captive diet should include nectar, insects, and other protein sources as well as limited amounts of fruits and vegetables. The quantity of food provided should be limited to 15% to 20% of body weight, depending on energy requirements associated with age, ambient temperature, breeding condition, and enclosure size.[17]
- Body weight should be monitored regularly and the quantity fed adjusted accordingly.

- Body condition can be assessed by palpation of the gliding membrane, which should be thin and flexible, not rounded with fat. Normal feces are elongated, firm ellipses 12 mm × 4 mm and dark-brown to black, and are sometimes joined by hairs ingested when the animal grooms.[12]
- The diet should be offered in fresh portions in the evening.

In groups, some individuals may emerge early to consume more than their share of food. Multiple feedings stations in the enclosure should be provided, or obese, dominant animals can be locked in the nest box until subordinate animals have fed.

- A portion of the diet should consist of sources of fruit sugars, preferably in the form of a sap or nectar. Sources include fresh nectar, maple syrup, honey, and artificial nectar products.
- Examples of commercial products include prepared lory diets and Gliderade (Avico, Fallbrook, CA).
- Gum Arabic (acacia) can be purchased as a powder, mixed into a thick paste, and used to simulate native gums: it can be used in holes in branches and on surfaces, with insects or bits of fruit stuck to it for enrichment and foraging.[13] Discussion of gum acacia is similar to the Australian acacia sp. Gum acacia has been shown to contain 1% dry weight calcium (Ca) and offsets the lack of Ca in arthropods eaten by the Senegal bush baby. In this respect, it would be valuable to know if mineral content of gums is similar between African and Australian acacia, such that gum Arabic might provide a suitable, available substitute feed for gliders.[15]
- Various commercial diets for sugar gliders and insectivores are available and may be included as a part of the diet.
- Leafy green vegetables provide a source of fiber and some vitamins. Sugar gliders accept a wide variety of other foods, including fruits, vegetables, nuts, and seeds (sunflower, pumpkin), but these should be offered in very limited quantities.
- Fruit juices and strained baby foods can be offered if they are free of preservatives, but they are not as appropriate as the nectar-based formulas. Because these foods are not a significant component of the natural diet, they should constitute less than 10% of the captive diet.
- Sprinkle a broad-spectrum vitamin and mineral supplement with a good Ca supply on the food daily.[9,13,18]

Contrary to nutritional needs observed in the wild, much of the information found in lay publications lists fruits and vegetables as a major portion of the captive diet.

- Fruit-based diets are harmful to captive sugar gliders because they provide inadequate protein and Ca and predispose animals to osteoporosis and periodontal disease.
- Although sugar gliders readily accept fruits, nuts, and grains, these are not a substantial part of their natural diet.

Sugar gliders do not require particularly high-protein diets, and excessive protein may, in fact, be detrimental to overall health; refining amino acid balance and overall level is critical for understanding and providing optimal protein nutrition.

- In this respect, use of a properly balanced dry or canned commercial product that also includes vitamins and minerals essential for other omnivorous species (ie, dogs or primates) is superior to protein sources comprising unsupplemented animal products, such as meat, eggs, and insects.[15]

Leadbeater's diet has been recommended as a base mixture for many sugar glider diets. This diet is an artificial nectar mix originally formulated for Leadbeater's possums (*Gymnobelideus leadbeati*). Leadbeater's recipe is listed in **Box 1**.

- The mixture is kept refrigerated until served, with the unused refrigerated portion discarded after 2 to 3 days. The mixture can be kept longer if frozen.
- The original Leadbeater's recipe is often modified by individuals with adjustments usually being made for palatability rather than nutritional content. Several modified versions are found on the Internet, such as Bourbon's Modified Leadbeater's Diet and the High Protein Wombaroo Diet (Wombaroo, Adelaide, SA, Australia). These diets should be scrutinized closely because they have not undergone thorough nutritional dietary trials and analysis.

A detailed study to investigate basic nutritional parameters was conducted comparing 3 commonly fed captive diets in sugar gliders.[16]
The following 3 diets were tried:

- Diet A: 15 g insectivore fare (Reliable Protein Products, Phoenix, AZ);
- Diet B: 15 g soaked dry test extrusion (the dry extrusion was soaked in water to improve palatability as a ratio of 1 part dry kibble [Eight in One Pet Products, Hauppauge, NY] to 2 parts water); or
- Diet C: 15 g homemade formulation, Bourbon's Modified Leadbeater's diet (for the most current version of this recipe description, see http://www.sugargliders.org/gliderinfo/diets/bml.htm). Fifteen grams of frozen mixed vegetables (peas, corn, and carrots) and assorted fresh fruit or frozen berries were offered with each treatment.
- Diet A was supplemented daily with 1 g of a 1:1 mix of RepCal Ca supplement (nonphosphorus with vitamin D_3; Rep-Cal Research Labs, Los Gatos, CA) and Vionate powder (Gimborn Pet Specialties, LLC, Atlanta, GA) added to the fruit. In addition, diet A contained 4 protein supplements each week. One teaspoon 1:1 of chopped boiled chicken and Special K (Kellogg's, Battle Creek, MI) cereal mix moistened with apple juice was added on 2 days and 10 mealworms were added on 2 other days.
- Diet B was supplemented daily with 0.5 g of Frugivore Salad Supplement (HMS Diets, Bluffton, IN) on the produce mixture, and 5 mealworms were added 4 times a week.
- Diet C was supplemented with 5 mealworms added 4 times a week. As for the basal diet, the soaked kibble diet (diet B) appeared to be consumed to the greatest extent, followed by diet C, and last, insectivore fare. Vegetables were the least preferred. The analysis of the chemical composition of diets offered to and eaten by sugar gliders is shown in **Table 4**.

The conclusion of the authors was that none of the 3 diets tested appear to contain the optimal balance for meeting the nutritional needs of sugar gliders, but the information obtained did provide further insight into the dietary requirements.

- Ca deficiencies can lead to tetany and have been reported in gliders. These deficiencies have been linked with diets high in fruits and insects, preferred food items that can be poor sources of Ca, and hence, the need for supplementing this mineral. However, one must be careful in supplying Ca to maintain nutrient balance. The optimal ratio of Ca and phosphorus (P) is 1:1 to 2:1, at least as much Ca as P and, optimally, twice as much Ca as P.
- In these diets, only diet B (soaked kibble diet) contained the optimal Ca:P ratio, and it was marginally optimal at 1:1.

Box 1
Diets suggested for sugar gliders

1. 50:50 Leadbeater's mixture: insectivore diet (Reliable Protein Products, Mazuri; see **Table 7**) Leadbeater's:

   - 150 mL warm water, 150 mL honey, 1 shelled hard-cooked egg, 25 g baby cereal, 1 teaspoon vitamin/mineral supplement. Mix warm water and honey. In a separate container, blend egg until homogenized, gradually adding honey/water, then vitamin powder, then baby cereal, blending thoroughly after each addition until smooth. Keep refrigerated until served.

2. Chicago Zoo:

   1 teaspoon-sized piece each, chopped: apple, carrot, sweet potato, banana, leaf lettuce, $^1/_2$ hard-cooked egg yolk, 1 tablespoon Nebraska Feline diet (or other good-quality zoo feline diet such as Mazuri; see **Table 7**), 1 dozen mealworms.

3. Taronga Zoo (feeds 2 gliders):

   3 g apple, 3 g banana/corn, 1.5 g dog kibble, 1 teaspoon fly pupae (mealworms substituted here), 3 g grapes/kiwi fruit, 2 teaspoons Leadbeater's mix, 4 g orange with skin, 2 g pear, 2 g cantaloupe/melon/papaya, 3 g sweet potato. On Wednesdays: feed day-old chick large insects (crickets substituted here), when available.

4. Booth diet:

   Offer a total of 15%–20% of body weight daily. Select one diet (a or b) from each of the following groups (1, 2, and 3) every day. Rotation between the diets is recommended but not necessary. Animals will benefit from a regular supply of vitamin/mineral-enriched insects.

   Group 1

   a. Insects: 75% moths, crickets, beetles; 25% fly pupae, mealworms

   b. Meat mix: commercial small carnivore or insectivore mix

   Group 2

   a. Nectar mix: 337.5 g fructose, 337.5 g sucrose (brown sugar), 112.5 g glucose made up to 2 L with warm water; commercially available mixes have some vitamin/mineral additives and may be used.

   b. Dry lorikeet mix: 900 g rolled oats, 225 g wheat germ, 225 g brown sugar, 112.5 g glucose, 112.5 g raisins or sultanas

   Group 3

   a. Fruit and vegetables: select for diced apple, nectarine, melon, grapes, raisins, sultanas, figs, tomato, sweet corn kernels, sweet potato, beans, shredded carrot, butternut pumpkin

   b. Greens: mixed sprouts, leaf/romaine lettuce, broccoli, parsley; with a vitamin/mineral supplement at the manufacturer's directions

5. Dierenfeld Diet 1: an adequate sample daily diet:

   5 g dry or 10 g semi-moist cat food, 5 g berries, 5 g citrus, 5 g other fruit, 5 g sweet potato, 1 g mealworm (or other vertebrates, such as grasshoppers, moths, fly pupae, crickets, optional)

   Such a diet provides 126 kJ energy, 21% crude protein (1750 mg), 0.77% Ca, 0.64% P, vitamin D 1.1 IU/g with this particular dry (generic) cat food

6. Dierenfeld Diet 2: blend into a slurry:

   12 g chopped, mixed fruit (any type, <10% citrus), 2.5 g cooked, chopped vegetables, 10 g peach or apricot nectar, 5.5 g ground, dry, low-iron bird diet, 1 g mealworm (or other invertebrates as above; optional). This diet provides 159 kJ energy, 17% crude protein (1550 mg), 0.61% Ca, 0.44% P, and vitamin D 0.9 IU/kg.

Data from Refs.[10,12,13,15,16,18]

Table 4
Chemical composition (nutrients on a dry matter basis) of diets offered to and eaten by sugar gliders, n = 3 animals per treatment

Diet	% Protein	% Fat	% Ca	% P
Diet A: Offered	25.6	6.6	1.3	0.2
Eaten	23.5	5.6	2.0	0.2
Diet B: Offered	25.9	13.8	0.7	0.7
Eaten	25.6	13.5	0.7	0.7
Diet C: Offered	18.6	7.6	2.9	0.4
Eaten	19.0	8.8	3.5	0.5

- Diet A, as prepared, contained 6.5 times more Ca than P, and as eaten, 10 times more Ca than P.
- Similarly, diet C contained 7 to 8 times more Ca than P. Although absolute Ca requirements of sugar gliders are unknown, based on other animals, a value between 0.5% and 1% of dry matter is anticipated for this species, with a dietary P requirement between 0.2% and 0.5%.
- Diet B appears too high in P relative to Ca, whereas diets A and C both appear too low.
- Bone density checks through radiographic examination would be one means of evaluating whether these diets may have affected bone quality though imbalanced Ca:P ratios. Radiographs appeared normal in all gliders during the course of this investigation.[16]

They did find the following:

1. Young, healthy male gliders appear to require between 105 kJ per day and 147 kJ per day—not many calories.
2. Total protein (as nitrogen) was apparently not limiting in any of the diets, but quality may have been marginal, particularly in diet C (evidenced by weight loss).
3. Diets currently being fed to captive sugar gliders are highly digestible; however, additional comparisons to determine digestibility of natural diets, especially gums, to target optimal nutrient levels are required; and
4. Evidence of mineral and vitamin imbalances in commonly fed diets, especially vitamin D and iron, which may be impacting health, need to be investigated further.
   - One discussion item was also needed to identify whether gliders have the enzyme for making their own vitamin C as do many animals. If so, excess dietary supplementation may not be warranted and may actually contribute to iron overload.
   - Still also needing investigation is blood carrier and storage proteins for iron saturation of transferring and ferritin in this species.
   - Still needed to know are the effects of gums on the gut health. They have a huge cecum for fermenting soluble fiber and really are not given much opportunity to do so with current feeding practices. The effects of different, simple and complex sugars on gut health, microbiology, and overall physiology need to be investigated in more detail.[16]

FEEDING RECOMMENDATIONS

- Adult captive sugar gliders weighing 130 g require between approximately 76 kJ and 147 kJ (18–35 kcal) per day to meet maintenance energy requirements, containing less than 500 mg crude protein, depending on protein quality.[15,16]

- Fresh food should be offered daily in as-fed amounts, approximately 25% to 30% of body weight (wet basis containing approximately 75% water), or approximately 7% to 9% dry-matter intake.
- As a broad rule of thumb, a mixture of one part dry or semi-moist commercial product to 2 parts (by weight) mixed fruits and vegetables (three-quarter fruits, one-quarter vegetables) meets sugar glider's energy and protein needs.
- If animals are particularly active or are at increased physiologic stages (growth, reproduction), then increase the portion of commercial product, rather than the produce, up to one-part dry or semi-moist to one-part produce. If the basal diet is nutritionally complete and consumed in these proportions, there should be little need for additional supplementation.
- All foods should be high quality; consumption of preferred food items (insects, fruits) should be closely monitored and restricted, such that consumption of balanced calories from the commercial portion of the diet is assured.

Box 1 lists several diets that have been fed successfully to sugar gliders. A diet should be chosen and fed in its entirety. The diet should be offered in fresh portions in the evening. Commercially available adult insects should be fed a Ca-rich insect diet for several days before being offered. Larval forms should be kept to a minimum. Chop the pieces together so that the gliders cannot pick out only their favorite items. No commercial diets seem totally adequate, but long-term nutritional studies are still pending.

- From a crude-protein perspective, dry dog, avian, or primate foods lower in protein (approximately 15%–25% dry basis) than cat foods (approximately 30%–45% protein) could be used to meet the protein requirements of sugar gliders.
- Fruits and vegetables can be frozen and thawed; however, canned fruits packed in syrup or processed vegetables should not be used.
- Fresh produce is preferred, particularly fruits and vegetables that contain more Ca than P (ie, berries, citrus, figs, papaya, or flower blossoms).
- Minimize use of fruits with inverse Ca:P ratios (ie, grapes, bananas, apples, pears, melon). Information on mineral balance can be found on the United States Department of Agriculture Nutrient Database (http://www.nal.usda.gov/fnic/foodcomp/search).
- Treats also must be carefully controlled to prevent obesity. Three grams (one-half teaspoon) of unsupplemented applesauce, for example, provides up to 7% of daily calculated energy needs for a 130-g sugar glider. Such treats should be factored in as part of the daily total dietary produce allotment.[15]

MACROPODS

Macropods are herbivorous foregut fermenters with a chambered stomach.

- The stomach comprises a sacciform forestomach, tubiform forestomach, hind-stomach, and pylorus. Microbial fermentation of ingested material occurs in the enlarged forestomach, with hydrochloric acid and pepsinogen being secreted in the hind stomach.
- A cecum is present but is not considered a major site of fermentation.[14]
- Merycism occurs in some macropods and is defined as regurgitation and reingestion (but no remastication) of forestomach contents. The kangaroo releases virtually no methane gas during eructation and exhalation due to the hydrogen byproduct of fermentation being converted into acetate, which is used for additional energy.

- The major advantages of foregut fermentation are the degradation of plant toxins and the ability to extract nutrition for poor-quality forage.
- Detailed physiologic and anatomic studies suggest that the macropod forestomach has more in common with the equine colon than the bovine forestomach.[2,14,19]

Macropods can be loosely grouped into 3 main classifications based on dietary preference:

1. Primary browsers
2. Primary grazers
3. Intermediate browser/grazer grade.
   - In general, the larger species tend to be primarily grazers, whereas the smaller species are primarily browsers. The Tammar and Bennett's wallabies are classified as intermediate grades, with wild-type diet being short grass, forbs, and bushes. The red kangaroo (*Macropus rufus*) is an example of a grazer (grass, forbs).[19]

ENERGY METABOLISM

On average, marsupials have a lower metabolism rate than their eutherian counterparts.

- The BMR of most marsupials decreases between 65% and 74% (mean, 70%) of the calculated BMR for a eutherian mammal of equal weight, with macropods ranging from 57% to 88%.
- This lower BMR results in lower average body temperatures and an overall decreased caloric requirement when compared with eutherians.
- The maintenance energy requirement for marsupials is usually 150% to 250% of the BMR, with larger marsupials having a maintenance energy requirement in the lower end of the range.[2,19]

The primary source of energy for macropods is short-chain fatty acids produced by microbes through fermentation.

- Most short-chain fatty acids are produced and absorbed in the forestomach, with production and absorption highest in the sacciform region.
- The cecum and proximal colon also serve as a secondary site of microbial fermentation.
- Short-chain fatty acids can lower the forestomach pH from approximately 8.0 in a fasting animal to approximately 5.0 in a recently fed animal.
- The types and proportions of short-chain fatty acids are similar to those produced in the rumen of domestic species.
- Like in ruminants, large proportions of acetic acid are converted to butyric acid, the principal short-chain fatty acids used by the forestomach epithelium for energy.
- Byproducts of this reaction are ketone bodies, especially acetoacetate, which can be further oxidized by other tissues.
- Unlike ruminants, however, in which this ketogenic activity occurs throughout the squamous epithelial lining of the rumen, ketogenic activity in macropods is restricted to the cardiac glandular mucosa.[2,20]

Microbial fermentation also results in production of ammonia, which serves as the primary nitrogen source for microbial protein synthesis.

- The ability of microbes to break down proteins, other microbes, and nonprotein nitrogen sources into ammonia allows macropods to use different nitrogen sources of varying quality. During periods of nitrogen shortage when ingesting a low-protein diet, macropods are able to recycle endogenously produced urea into the gut to be used as a nitrogen source instead of excreting it in the urine. Gases produced by forestomach fermentation are primarily carbon dioxide and hydrogen. Methane is also produced, especially during active eating, but at lower levels compared with ruminants.[2,20]
- Soluble sugars are rapidly digested and absorbed in the sacciform forestomach. This process results in little disaccharidase activity in the small intestines, because few digestible carbohydrates ever reach this location before they are broken down by microbes and absorbed.
- Similar to sheep, there is minimal glucose uptake into the liver. Instead, the liver continuously produces and releases glucose into the blood through gluconeogenesis, which occurs postprandially and during fasting.
- Macropods exhibit considerable tolerance to hypoglycemia induced by intravenous injections of insulin; however, they are much less tolerant of hyperglycemia.[2,19,20]

The tubular flow of ingesta through the macropod forestomach results in a shorter retention time.

- One disadvantage to this system is that digestibility of the ingesta is lower compared with ruminants of similar size.
- An advantage of this system is that dietary fiber continues to move through the forestomach regardless of fiber length and size.
- In ruminants, the rumen retains fiber particles until they are degraded to a certain size, which prolongs digestion and results in greater rumen fill and decreased dietary intake. High-fiber diets can limit food intake in ruminants.
- Dietary intake in macropods depends less on fiber content. Smaller macropods (with larger sacciform forestomachs) are more affected by dietary fiber than the larger grazing macropods.[19]

In captivity, macropods should be given a diet that best approximates the forage consumed by wild members of a given species. Access to high-quality grass pasture is recommended, especially for grazing species (**Fig. 6**). Nontoxic browse items also can be offered to provide variety and mimic natural behaviors. For many species, providing fresh limbs with leaves and bark allows macropods to consume the leaves

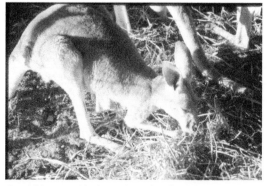

Fig. 6. Macropods should be provided good quality fresh hay.

and strip the bark, which also provides behavioral enrichment. An example of diet composition is listed in **Table 5**. **Table 6** lists micronutrient composition needed by macropods.[19]

Basic captive diets mimic those fed to ungulates.

- Items are given in lower quantities on a per weight basis, however, because of lower metabolism rates of macropods.
- If overfed, some species (especially smaller ones) are predisposed to obesity.
- Good quality grass hay is recommended ad libitum for all species, especially if not kept on a grass pasture.
- Quality is important because coarse, sharp, or abrasive food items (eg, oat awns, stalky hay, hay contaminated with thorny plants) can cause oral trauma and provide an avenue for secondary bacterial infections that lead to soft tissue infections, dental lesions, and osteomyelitis (commonly but controversially referred to as "lumpy jaw"). Lucerne (alfalfa) can also be offered.
- Food items should not be too soft either (eg, bread), because soft foods do not adequately toughen the oral mucosa or wear the teeth to allow molar progression.
- Macropods are susceptible to toxoplasmosis from ingesting food items contaminated with infected cat feces.
- Contamination of hay from barn cats at the hay storage location has been implicated as the source of toxoplasmosis outbreaks in several zoologic collections.
- It is recommended that food items be fed elevated from the ground (eg, in a hay rack, elevated bowl, or trough feeder) to prevent contamination with feces and reduce the transmission of parasites. Food containers should be cleaned daily and regularly disinfected.
- To reduce food competition and aggression, multiple feeding areas are recommended when macropods are kept in a group.[21]

Box 2 lists a suggested diet for captive macropods. Pelleted rations are also recommended in moderation. Several commercially available pellets formulated specifically for macropods are available and are listed in **Table 7**.

- Vegetables can be offered in small amounts, and fruits can be used only as an occasional treat. These produce items must be restricted to a small proportion

Table 5	
Macropod pelleted diet example: pelleted maintenance diet for grazing kangaroos	
Component	**Inclusion (% of Air-Dried Feed)**
Milled straw	50.0
Chopped alfalfa (Lucerne) hay	47.0
NaCl	0.75
CaH_2PO_4	0.75
$CaCO_3$	0.75
$MgSO_4$	0.12
KCl	0.22
$NaSO_3$	0.21
Micronutrient mix	0.20

Data from Hume ID, Barboza PS. Designing artificial diets for captive marsupials. In: Fowler ME, editor. Zoo and wild animal medicine. 3rd edition. Philadelphia: WB Saunders; 1993. p. 281–8.

Table 6
Micronutrient mix for grazing marsupials

Component	Amount (/kg of Air-Dried Feed)
Fe	10 mg
Co	1 mg
Mn	58 mg
Zn	50 mg
I	0.7 mg
Se	2 ng
Vitamin A	12,000 IU
Vitamin D	2400 IU
Vitamin E	30 IU
Vitamin B1	2 mg
Vitamin B2	6 mg
Vitamin B6	2 mg
Vitamin B12	20 ng
Pantothenic acid	5.5 mg
Niacin	26 mg
Choline	200 mg
Vitamin K	0.6 mg
Biotin	320 ng
Folic acid	0.4 mg

of the diet, however, because they contain higher levels of simple sugars and carbohydrates and are easily fermentable, possibly leading to gastrointestinal and dental problems.

- Sweet feed mixes should not be used for the same reasons.
- Items such as bread, peanut butter, jam, and other sweet treats may be helpful in getting a macropod to take medications, but they should not be a regular part of the diet (**Fig. 7**).

Box 2
Suggested diet for macropods

- Free-choice grass or Timothy hay or pasture for grazing
- Daily concentrate herbivore pellet to provide energy, microminerals and macrominerals, with vitamin E
- Pelleted feed approximately 25% daily diet
- Complete marsupial feeds, such as Mazuri Kangaroo Pellet (PMI Nutrition International, Inc, Brentwood, MO)
- Nonmarsupial herbivore pelleted feed (Mazuri Lagomorph, Equid, Oxbow Rabbit), must be supplemented with Vitamin E at 200–600 mg/d for adult macropods.
- Treats: small amounts of domestic produce (vegetables, occasional fruit). Domestic produce is high in carbohydrates and generally low in fiber.

Data from Refs.[9,10,17]

Table 7
Guaranteed analysis of selected commercial diets

Diet	Protein %	Fat %	Fiber %	Form	Product Size
5Z88 Mazuri Exotic canine diet	28.5	18.0	4.0	Extruded particle	3/8″ × 5/16″
5661 Mazuri Equid maintenance	13.0	2.0	15.0	Pellet	5/32″ × $\frac{1}{2}$″
5MK8 Mazuri Insectivore diet	28.0	12.0	13.0	Extruded particle	1/16″ × 1/16″
5Z88 Mazuri Kangaroo/wallaby	15.0	5.0	10.0	Extruded pellets	3/8″ × 3/16″
5652 Mazuri Lagomorph diet	16.0	2.0	18.0	Pellet	5/32″ × $\frac{3}{4}$″
5635 Mazuri Omnivore zoo feed "A"	25.0	6.0	5.0	Extruded biscuit	$\frac{1}{2}$″ × 1″
Fox reproduction diet, Milk Specialties Company	35.0	13.0	4.5	Extruded pellet	1/4″ diameter
Insectivore fare, Reliable Protein Products	20.0	6.0	6.0	Soft pellets	1/4″ diameter
Oxbow Pet Products Essentials Adult Rabbit	14.0	2.0	25–29	Pellet	$\frac{1}{4}$″ × $\frac{1}{2}$″ approximately

Data from Refs.[22–24]

- Carrots can be offered as treats.
- Salt blocks are recommended for the species commonly kept in captivity as a source of electrolytes and minerals.
- Fresh, clean water should be offered daily to all macropods. Although some species are drought-tolerant, captive diets usually contain less moisture than wild forages, which increases the captive animal's need for water intake. Plants toxic to domestic herbivores or chemically treated items should not be fed.[19,21]

Vitamin E is an antioxidant required by macropods to prevent myopathy, or white muscle disease.

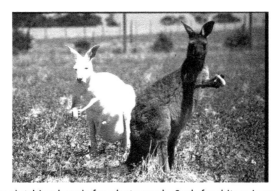

Fig. 7. Kangaroos clutching bagels for photograph. Such food item is not recommended.

- Hind limb weakness that progressed to paralysis, muscle wasting, and death was described in captive Quokkas (*Setonix brachyurus*) fed a commercial sheep pellet.
- Smaller enclosure sizes were found to increase the requirement of vitamin E because of the additional stress of overcrowding.
- Myopathy, however, was prevented with vitamin E supplementation regardless of enclosure size.
- In most species of animals, selenium can be used as an antioxidant substitute in place of vitamin E to prevent myopathy, but selenium supplementation alone was found to be ineffective in preventing myopathy Tammar wallabies.
- Vitamin E supplementation is recommended for all macropods. The amount required will vary based on the vitamin E content of the diet ingredients. Feeding large amounts of varied natural browse may reduce the need for vitamin E supplementation.[19]

Table 7 lists commercial diets mentioned in this article.[22–24]

VIRGINIA OPOSSUM

Virginia opossums are true omnivores.[10,17,25]

- The diet eaten by free-ranging opossums includes any and all green and yellow vegetables, grass, fruit, carrion, snails, slugs, worms, insects including flies, earwigs, roaches, amphibians, eggs, crayfish, and fish.[10,25,26]
- They may also eat birds but rarely eat the entire carcass.
- In captivity, they can be fed a varied diet that includes good-quality dog and/or cat foods, various vegetables, fruits, an occasional egg, supplemental Ca and vitamin A, live foods (such as crickets, slugs, mealworms), and yogurt. Opossums are particularly indiscriminate and will consume nearly any food offered.[17] Formulations have been developed for different stages of life.
- The gastrointestinal morphology is consistent with that of many other mammalian omnivores.
- The dental formula is 5/4, 1/1, 3/3, 4/4.
- The salivary glands include large mandibular and smaller parotid and sublingual glands.
- The distal esophagus has raised, transverse rugae and comprises smooth muscle fibers.
- The opossum's distal esophagus, pylorus, and ileocecal junction have been studied extensively, because the smooth muscle arrangements in these areas closely resemble that of humans.[27]
- Virginia opossums have a simple, globular stomach; most of the gastric mucosa is composed of fundic glands.
- Pyloric glands, and a narrow ridge of cardiac glands, exist near the esophageal-gastric border.
- Like most placental mammals, opossums have enteroendocrine cells lining portions of the gastrointestinal tract. These cells, in addition to endocrine cells in the pancreas, aid in secreting peptides that control various digestive functions, such as gastric acid secretion, pancreatic secretion of electrolytes and enzymes, and contraction of the gall bladder.
- In the stomach, 90% of the enteroendocrine cells are located in the pyloric region and secrete a variety of hormones, such as gastrin, gastric-inhibitory peptide, secretin, cholecystokinin, and pancreozymin.[27]

- The Brunner's glands secrete their products into mucosal depression located on the duodenal wall.
- The cecum is simple, conical, and approximately 20% to 40% of the total body length.
- Distal to the cecum, the colon is mobile because of its simple, loose mesenteric attachment.

ADULT OPOSSUM NUTRITION

In a study of opossums in New York, analysis of the stomach contents of 187 road-killed opossums showed that the average opossum diet consisted of 18% fruit, 17.2% amphibians, 14.2% mammals, 13.4% insects, 6.6% grass, 5.4% worms, 5.3% reptiles, 5% birds, 4.8% carrion, and 6.7% other items. Another study showed that stomach contents of road-killed opossums in Portland, Oregon consisted of 27% mammals, 11% leaf litter, 10% fruits, seeds, and bulbs, 10% gastropods, 9% garbage, 9% earthworms, 9% pet food, 8% grass and green leaves, 3% insects, 3% birds, and 1% unidentified animal tissue. Both studies looked at stomach rather than fecal content because fecal analysis reveals food items that readily pass through the gastrointestinal system and may not account for more digestible food items.[27]

Many adult diet variations exist. Maintaining the proper Ca:P ratio and avoiding high fat meals should be a priority.

- Virginia opossums need an increased Ca component in their diet, especially as juveniles and young adults, that is typically consumed as whole prey and egg-shells. As these items are usually minimized in captive rations, a human pediatric Ca supplement should be offered daily until full maturity.
- Milk products should be fed scarcely, as they are lactose-based; this sugar is poorly tolerated by the marsupial digestive system.[17]

Suggested diets for adult opossums are listed in **Table 8**.

VITAMINS

- If given an appropriately balanced diet, healthy opossums do not need vitamin supplementation.
- When appropriate diets are given, vitamin deficiencies are uncommon, and the risk of health problems associated with over-supplementation can be avoided.
- Vitamin D deficiencies are uncommon in opossums because they, like other crepuscular mammals, are highly efficient at producing vitamin D_3 (cholecalciferol, the active form of vitamin D) in the skin, compared with diurnal mammals that require exposure to sunlight to active vitamin D. If vitamin D must be supplemented, only products that contain cholecalciferol should be given. Over-supplementation with vitamin D can lead to demineralization of bone and mineralization of soft tissues and should be avoided. A single dose of vitamin D_3 may be stored in the body for as long as 6 months.[27]

Opossums usually do not need to be supplemented with vitamin A, which is fat soluble and derived from carotenoids found in plants.

- It is formed in the intestinal epithelium of most animals and stored in the liver. Vitamin A is essential for maintenance and growth of surface epithelium, eye pigmentation, and bones.
- Over-supplementation can prevent bone formation and stimulate bone resorption.

Table 8
Suggested diets for adult opossums (choose one and use in entirety)

Diet 1	Diet 2	Diet 3

Evening:
    112.5 g chopped mixed vegetables (not corn, peas)
    15 g mixed chopped fruits (not citrus)
    15 mL nonfat yogurt
    56 g insectivore or omnivore zoo pelleted diet
    3–4 times a week:
        0.25 hard-cooked egg OR 15 g canned salmon OR 56 g cooked tofu
    50 mg pharmaceutical grade calcium carbonate or Ca gluconate powder: mix into the vegetables/fruit at least 3 times a week
    Children's multiple vitamin can be given 1–2 times a week as a treat
Other treats: 1 king mealworm OR 1–2 Ca gut-loaded crickets OR 3–4 mealworms: 2–4 times a week
Morning:
    56 g dry cat food, insectivore, omnivore kibble
	Evening:
	    56 g dry dog food, insectivore, or omnivore kibble
	    56 g meat-based canned dog or cat food mixed into the kibble
	    56 g mixed fruit
	    56 g mixed vegetables
	    Calcium carbonate should be sprinkled on fruits/vegetables and mixed in
	Morning:
	    56 g dry cat, insectivore, or omnivore kibble
	    Treats: Once daily
	    5 mL nonfat fruit yogurt OR 1 children's multiple vitamin OR 1 king mealworm OR 1–2 Ca-loaded crickets OR 3–4 mealworms
		6 tablespoons of a dry, high-quality cat food
		1/2 cup of small vegetable chunks
		2–3 teaspoons of fruit
		7 tablespoons of a high-quality canned dog food
		Several earthworms
		1 hard-cooked egg with shell
		1 whole mouse (approximately 30 g)
		Feed once a day; unlimited fresh water

Data from Refs.[10,25,27]

- Supplemental vitamin A should be given only when deficiencies are suspected, and doses should be carefully monitored, because hypervitaminosis A can contribute to metabolic bone disease.[27]

The most common nutritional diseases seen in pet Virginia opossums are nutritional secondary hyperparathyroidism caused by Ca:P imbalances or deficiency of Ca, obesity, and dental disease.[25]

Food consumption required is about 150 to 200 g per day per adult. To prevent obesity, dry food may need to be limited and fed as meals rather than ad libitum. Commercial dry hedgehog/insectivore diet is being used in place of dry dog/cat food. No feeding trials have been done, but the commercial insectivore and omnivore diets are generally lower in fat than the dog/cat foods, which may be advantageous for controlling weight.[10] Suggested diets are listed in **Table 8** (**Fig. 8**).

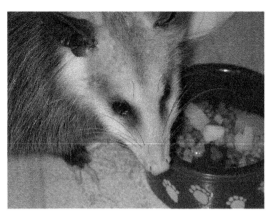

Fig. 8. Adult opossum with diet showing insectivore pellets and chopped vegetables.

SHORT-TAILED OPOSSUM

Wild short-tailed opossums eat small prey (mice, insects), fruit, grains, and carrion.[9]

As laboratory animals, they have been maintained and bred with success using a commercial pelleted fox food (Reproduction Diet, Nutritionally Complete Fox Food Pellets; Milk Specialties Products, New Holstein, WI).[9] It has a fat content of 10% dry weight and cholesterol content of 0.15% of dry weight. Opossums fed a diet containing 18.8% fat with cholesterol content of 0.71% in genetically predisposed animals developed hypercholesterolemia.[28,29] They are used as an animal model of dietary-induced hyperlipidemia and hypercholesterolemia. They have also been successfully maintained in the laboratory on a diet of Purina Cat Chow (Nestle Purina, St Louis, MO) fed ad libitum.[30] Supplements have been insects and pinky mice. Usually the meal is fed in the evening. Live foods are let loose in the cage. Fruit can be placed on branches to encourage foraging and exercise (**Fig. 9**).[10] Suggested diets for the short-tailed opossum are listed in **Table 9**.

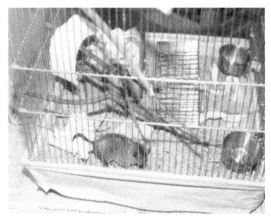

Fig. 9. Short-tailed opossum with grapes placed on branches for foraging.

Table 9	
Suggested diets for the short-tailed opossum	
Diet 1 (Adapted from the National Zoo, Washington, DC)	**Diet 2**

5 g of blended meat mixture comprising:
  225 g chopped, cooked lean meat (horse or beef)
  1 hard-cooked egg
  15 g wheat germ flakes
  10 g powdered milk
  2.5 g powdered multivitamin/mineral supplement
This mixture is supplemented daily with:
  1-cm cube of fresh fruit (kiwi, orange, apple, grape, banana)
  1-cm cube of commercial marmoset diet
  1 or 2 Ca gut-loaded crickets, 6 small mealworms OR 2 king mealworms OR 10 small mealworms. Note: adult insects are more nutritious than larval forms.
	5 g commercial insectivore diet (hedgehog dry kibble, zoo insectivore pellet diets)
	2.5 g cooked meat (turkey, chicken, beef, deboned fish) sprinkled with powdered multivitamin/mineral supplement
	1-cm cube of fresh fruit (kiwi, orange, apple, grape, banana) sprinkled with powdered multivitamin/mineral supplement
	1 or 2 Ca gut-loaded crickets
	1 large mealworm and 6 small mealworms OR 2 large mealworms OR 10 small mealworms. Note: adult insects are more nutritious than larval forms.
	In addition, 3–5 times a week:
	  1.25 g hard-cooked egg (chop white and yolk together, sprinkle with vitamin/mineral supplement)
	  1.25 g cottage cheese or skim-milk cheese

Data from Johnson-Delaney C. Marsupials. In: Meredith A, Johnson-Delaney C, editors. BSAVA manual of exotic pets. Fifth edition. A foundation manual. Quedgeley (United Kingdom): British Small Animal Veterinary Association; 2010. p. 103–26.

HAND-REARING

Marsupials are unique in that the embryo develops outside the uterus and depends on the teat secreting the appropriate milk for the age and maturation of the embryo. In captivity, this poses challenges and must approximate the natural process.

Macropods have 4 teats, although only one develops for each joey.

- As a survival strategy, some macropods have the capability of having 3 joeys at one time, each in a different stage of development.
- One joey can be out of the pouch but still nursing (young at foot, "YAF"), while another is developing in the pouch (pouch joey), and a third is waiting in utero as a result of embryonic diapauses.
- This occurrence can result in teats in 4 different stages of lactation: one undergoing regression from a previous joey, one for the YAF, one for the pouch joey, and one undeveloped teat for the joey yet to be born. The 2 teats that are actively lactating simultaneously produce milk of different compositions that are appropriate for each joey's stage of development.[19]

The role of the different milk during lactation has been studied. The mother progressively changes the composition of the major, and many minor, components of the milk.

- In contrast to eutherians, there is a far greater investment in development of the young during lactation and it is likely that many of the signals that regulate development of eutherian embryos in utero are delivered by the milk. This requires the coordinated development and function of the mammary gland because inappropriate timing of these signaling events may result in either limited or abnormal development of the young, and potentially a higher incidence of mature onset disease.

- Milk proteins play a significant role in these processes by providing timely presentation of signaling molecules and antibacterial protection for the young and the mammary gland at times when there is increased susceptibility to infection.[31]

Cross-fostering is rearing of young by a surrogate mother of a different taxon. In marsupials, this technique has been used to study lactation as well as pouch young growth and development. Data on cross-fostering are now available for 6 potoroid and 13 macropodid species.

- Studies have shown that female marsupials regulate milk composition and production irrespective of pouch young age, and that transfer of donor young to species with more immature or advanced mammary glands will result in a slowing or an acceleration of pouch young growth and development.
- The temperature and humidity within the pouch environment affects the duration of pouch life. Small pouch young tolerate short-term isolation from the pouch at a range of temperatures, provided high humidity is maintained throughout the period of isolation.
- Maintenance of pouch young at temperatures lower than those that occur in the pouch (23°C compared with 37°C) during isolation reduces the pouch young's BMR, oxygen consumption, and evaporative water loss and thus improves survival rates of very small pouch young.
- The success of these techniques in managing population genetics and accelerating breeding in donor species within the Macropodoidea are enhanced by post-partum estrus and mating after the removal of pouch young, and the reactivation and birth of the diapausing embryo.[32]

The effects on gastrointestinal maturation in tammar wallabies of providing younger pouch young with older-stage milk have been studied.

- There was a significant increase in pouch young weight when donor young were supplied with older-stage milk, possibly because of a higher concentration of lipid in milk from the more advanced mammary glands.
- However, no difference was found in stomach or small intestine development between young reared on the appropriate milk for age and those reared on milk for more advanced pouch young.[32]

The need for hand-rearing can occur as a result of health issues or death of the dam or if the dam throws the joey from the pouch as a result of stress. Artificial rearing of macropod joeys can be challenging. Commercial products for stage of development are available (Wombaroo; Perfect Pets Inc, Belleville, MI; **Box 3**).[33] Body measurements and not weight should be used along with species-specific growth charts to determine the joey's age. Artificial milk replacers designed for other species and whole milk from other species should not be used, because they often contain high levels of oligosaccharides (eg, lactose, sucrose). Because of previously described slower mechanism for digestion of these oligosaccharides in macropods, their use can result in severe problems, such as osmotic diarrhea, gastrointestinal bacterial overgrowth, and cataracts. More detailed information on hand-rearing macropods is available.[34]

METHODS

Orphaned joeys first need to be at a normal body temperature of 95 to 98.6°F (35–37°C) before feeding. The milk formulation should be chosen for the species and age class.

- A rule of thumb is to feed formula at 95°F (35°C).

Box 3
Artificial milk formulations specific for marsupials

Commercial marsupial formulations and nursing equipment:

Wombaroo Food Products, PO Box 151, Glen Osmond, SA 5064, Australia

US Distributors: Perfect Pets, Geoff Schrock, 23180 Sherwood Rd, Belleville, MI 48111; (734) 461-1362, Fax (734) 461-2858

Kangaroo Milk Replacer (for all macropods)

(<0.4, 0.4, 0.6, >0.7) key: less than 0.4, less than 40% pouch life complete

Possum Milk Replacer (for sugar gliders) (<0.8 for joeys with <80% pouch life complete; >0.8 for joeys with >80% pouch life complete)

Latex teats: STM: for small, in-pouch kangaroos, wallabies, possums

MTM: for in-pouch kangaroos, wallabies, koalas

TM: for out-of-pouch kangaroos, wallabies

SD: for possums, gliders

Biolac Milk Replacer for Marsupials

US Distributors: 675 Gooseberry Court, Lafayette, CO 80026; (303) 666-0924, Fax: (303) 666-0574. Australia: Geoff and Christine Smith, PO Box 93, Bonnyrigg, NSW 2177; 011 61 (02) 9823 9874

M100—early lactation milk

M150—mid lactation milk

M200—late lactation milk

M100-G—with galacto-oligosaccharides for furless joeys

T1—Long joey teat, hard or soft

T2—Long, fine teat, for very all orphans

T4—Short, fine teat, for sugar gliders

Data from Johnson-Delaney CA. Reproductive medicine of companion marsupials. Vet Clin North Am Exot Anim Pract 2002;5:537–53.

- Formulas should be made fresh, and utensils, teats, and bottles should be washed and sanitized after use.
- Unfurred animals are fed approximately every 2 to 3 hours and furred approximately every 4 hours. Frequency must be adjusted for the physical condition of the joey.
- Weak or dehydrated animals may require feedings every 2 hours.
- The amount of formula a joey should receive within a 24-hour period is related to its body weight and formula used. The rule of thumb is 10% to 20% of the body weight in formula every 24 hours, but no more than 20%.

Marsupial teats are shaped differently than those sold for domestic animals or humans. The hole in the teat must be small and can be made by piercing the teat several times with a hot needle. Alternatively, a syringe with a gastric feeding tube, feline urinary catheter, or intravenous catheter (needle removed) can be used to provide the small opening.

- Most joeys are best fed while in an artificial pouch, which can be fashioned from a sock, sweater, or towel.
- The environment needs to be dark, quiet, and without distractions. Covering the eyes with a hand during feeding may help.

- The joey should be weighed daily.
- When teeth have erupted and the joey is fully furred, small amounts of adult diet can be introduced.
- When the joey leaves the pouch for short periods, it should be provided adult food to investigate. Gradually decrease the formula feedings as the joey weans.
- Many companion marsupials will take formula or even plain water from a bottle long after weaning, which can facilitate the administration of medications and oral fluids if ever necessary.

SUGAR GLIDERS

Hand-rearing of sugar gliders has been documented.[13,35] Puppy Esbilac (Pet Ag, Hampshire, IL) has been used successfully to raise sugar gliders by one author, but there are recommendations to avoid Kitten Esbilac, goat's milk, cow's milk, or human milk replacer because of higher lactose contents than the canine formulation. This rearing recipe is included in **Box 4**.[33,35]

- Feed unfurred young every 1 to 2 hours, including throughout the night, and feed just-furred young every 4 hours.
- Gradually reduce the frequency to twice daily, then once daily, until the young are weaned.
- Guidelines for volume of milk to feed per day are shown in **Table 10** along with milestones and body weight with respect to age.[35]

Marsupial milk increases in energy at the time of pouch exit to provide for the young's increased energy demands of locomotion and thermoregulation. This change can be simulated by adding canola oil or rapeseed oil to the milk at the rate of 1 mL of oil per 20 mL of formula.[13]

- Juvenile sugar gliders usually lap readily from the tip of a syringe, or they can be taught to lap from a small plastic lid.
- At each feeding, measure and record milk intake.
- Measure body weight daily until the weight stabilizes, then weekly.
- Frequency of feeding and quantity of food can be adjusted to achieve a satisfactory growth rate.
- Start offering solids at about 100 days, at which time the young glider should weigh approximately 54 g, and wean at 130 days, when body weight is approximately 80 grams.[35]
- Pureed baby food with meat and vegetables or blended adult diet is a suitable starter food.[13]

Box 4
Puppy Esbilac formulation for sugar gliders

1 Scoop Puppy Esbilac powder (Pet Ag, Inc)

3 Scoops Pedialyte (initially, if dehydrated) or plain water (Abbott Laboratories, Abbott Park, IL)

Warm to body temperature, syringe feed one drop at a time every 2 h until furred.

Fully furred: feed every 3–4 hours

Once the eyes have opened, cease the night feedings.

At least twice daily or before feedings: stimulate urination and defecation by gently stroking the area of the cloaca and base of tail with a moistened cotton ball or swab.

Table 10			
Growth and development of young sugar gliders (*P breviceps*) from southeast Queensland (Guidelines for hand-rearing based on wild glider development)			
Age (d)	**Weight (g)**	**Feed (mL per day)**	**Milestones**
1	0.2	A few drops (author estimated for hand-rearing purposes)	Mouth and forelimbs most developed feature
20	0.8	A few drops (author estimated for hand-rearing purposes)	Ears free from head, papillae of mystacial vibrissae visible
35	2.0	1.0	Mystacial vibrissae (whiskers) erupt, ear pigmented. Realistic time to successfully hand-rear
40	3.0	1.5	Pigmentation starts on shoulder, eye slits present
60	12	3	Detaching from teat, fur emerging, dorsal stripe developing
70	20	4	Eyes open, fully furred, left in nest
80	35	6	Fur lengthens
90	44	7	
100	54	8	Emerging from nest, starting to eat solid foods
130	78		Weaned

Data from Barnes M. Sugar gliders. In: Gage LJ, editor. Hand-rearing wild and domestic animals. Ames (IA): Iowa State Press; 2002. p. 55–62.

MACROPODS

- An artificial formula has been used successfully. Wombaroo (Wombaroo Food Products, PO Box 151, Glen Osmond, SA, Australia) and Biolac (Biolac, Lafayette, CO) are commercially available marsupial milks with different concentrations of the major components to match the needs of joeys in different stages of development (see **Box 3**). These commercially available marsupial milks are low-lactose formulations.
- Start by diluting the formula with an oral rehydration electrolyte solution on the first 2 to 3 days to allow adjustment to the new formula. Half strength on day 1, two-thirds strength on day 2, three-quarter strength on day 3, and full-strength formula on day 4 is an example of a suitable regime.
- Unfurred joeys are fed every 1 to 2 hours.
- Recently furred young should be fed every 4 hours, and then the frequency of feeding should gradually be reduced to once or twice daily before weaning.
- Food intake should be measured and recorded at each feed. Simulate hand-raised young to urinate and defecate after each feed by gently wiping the cloaca with moistened cotton ball. Measure body weight daily until it has stabilized, then weekly.[33,34]

VIRGINIA OPOSSUMS

The National Opossum Society has published detailed infant diets, feeding instructions, and growth information for the Virginia opossum.[8] The basic formula can be made using either Esbilac or Multi-Milk (PetAg, Inc) at either 1:3 to 1:5 dilution with distilled water. Added to this is egg yolk, brewer's yeast, apple juice, or boysenberry low-fat yogurt.[36]

Another hand-rearing formulation has been used successfully to rear Virginia Opossums:

- Mix Puppy Esbilac, or Zoologic Milk Matrix 33/40 powder (all Pet Ag, Inc [1-800-323-0877 for product questions]) or Multi-Milk or Zoologic Milk Matrix 30/55 powder.
- One part Esbilac or Zoologic Milk Matrix 33/40 powder, $\frac{1}{2}$ part Multi-Milk or Zoologic Milk Matrix 30/55, 2 parts water. Mix by volume (ie, teaspoon, tablespoon, cup). If water quality is poor, use distilled water. Values shown are wet matter basis (percentage of mixed formula), 21.7% solids, 10.5% fat, 7.3% protein, 2.3% carbohydrates, 1.33 KCal/mL.[37]

By the time an opossum is 45 g, it can be taught to lap formula from a jar lid (**Fig. 10**). They will need to be encouraged.

- When the opossums are lapping regularly on their own, hand feeding can be reduced to once or twice a day or discontinued when they weigh 60 g or more. Formula needs to be thickened by adding ground or whole Purina Kitten Chow ("original formula" only; Nestle Purina PetCare, St. Louis, MO) that has been mixed with water.
- This mixture will be called "chow-pudding." Grind dry Purina Kitten Chow in a blender or food processor. Add a sufficient amount of water to give the chow a pudding-like consistency. Allow this to set in the refrigerator for approximately 10 minutes. It absorbs water faster when refrigerated.
- The whole consistency changes (there should not be any hard chunks). More water or more chow may be added to get the desired consistency. Thicken the formula with a small amount of the chow-pudding mix. It should resemble formula that has small particles of Kitten Chow throughout.
- As the joey becomes accustomed to the taste, increase the amount of the chow-pudding. Provide a lid of whole dry Purina Kitten Chow and another lid of Kitten Chow that has been soaked in water 5 to 10 minutes in whole form. Some animals eat the softer chow more readily. A shallow container of water should also be available. By the time the opossums weight 80 to 100 g, introduce the modified Jurgelski diet (**Box 5**). The diet composition is 33.2% solids, 3.3% fat, 13.9% protein, 11.2% carbohydrates equaling 21.2 KCal per tablespoon. Altering the amount of liver or using another brand of kitten food has and will

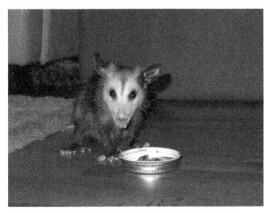

Fig. 10. Juvenile Virginia opossum eating out of a jar lid.

Box 5
Modified Jurgelski diet: precise measurements

Offer in the evening.

1 part ground, raw beef liver

9 parts Purina Kitten Chow pudding (ground dry chow mixed with enough water to give a pudding-like consistency)

To every cup of kitten chow pudding, add $^1/_4$ teaspoon pulverized calcium carbonate that equals 700–800 mg Ca per teaspoon.

Data from Taylor P. Opossums. In: Gage LJ, editor. Hand-rearing wild and domestic animals. Ames (IA): State Press; 2002. p. 45–54.

---

cause metabolic bone problems. The diet should be offered every evening. Some animals take longer than others to acquire a taste for this diet. When the opossum is consistently eating the modified Jurgelski diet, gradually add small quantities of various fresh fruits and vegetables (add one item at a time). Cut into bite-size pieces before offering them to the youngsters. The modified Jurgelski diet should constitute 90% of the total diet.[37]

In conclusion, much is known about the nutrition and dietary requirements of captive marsupials. The most important goal for clinicians is that there is enough information available from captive and field studies of the major species of marsupials (metabolic rates, effects of food habits, activity levels) to develop appropriate diets. Micronutrient components still need to be studied in many, but little should be left to guesswork, and diets should not be fed simply because the animal prefers certain food items. It is easy to overfeed captive marsupials.

REFERENCES

1. Hume ID. Omnivorous marsupials. In: Marsupial nutrition. Cambridge (United Kingdom): Cambridge Press; 1999. p. 76–124.
2. Hume ID. Foregut fermenters. In: Marsupial nutrition. Cambridge (United Kingdom): Cambridge Press; 1999. p. 205–60.
3. Hume ID. Nutritional ecology of kangaroos and wallabies. In: Marsupial nutrition. Cambridge (United Kingdom): Cambridge Press; 1999. p. 261–314.
4. Henry SR, Suckling GC. A review of the ecology of the sugar glider. In: Smith AP, Hume ID, editors. Possums and gliders. Chipping Norton (New South Wales): Surrey Beatty & Sons PTY Limited; 1984. p. 355–8.
5. Hume ID, Barboza PS. Designing artificial diets for captive marsupials. In: Fowler ME, editor. Zoo and wild animal medicine. 3rd edition. Philadelphia: WB Saunders; 1993. p. 281–8.
6. McMillan A, Coupland G, Chambers BK, et al. Determining the diet of tammar wallabies on Garden Island, Western Australia, using stable isotope analysis. In: Coulson G, Eldridge M, editors. Macropods: the biology of kangaroos, wallabies and rat-kangaroos. Collingwood (Victoria): CSIRO Publishing; 2010. p. 171–7.
7. The Opossum Base. Available at: http://opossumbase.org/. Accessed November 19, 2013.
8. The National Opossum Society. 2006. Available at: http://www.opossum.org. Accessed November 21, 2013.

9. Johnson-Delaney CA. Marsupials. In: Exotic companion handbook for veterinarians. Lake Worth (FL): Wingers Publishing; 1996. p. 1–52.

10. Johnson-Delaney C. Marsupials. In: Meredith A, Johnson-Delaney C, editors. BSAVA manual of exotic pets Fifth edition a foundation manual. Quedgeley (United Kingdom): British Small Animal Veterinary Association; 2010. p. 103–26.

11. Hume ID. Metabolic rates and nutrient requirements. In: Marsupial nutrition. Cambridge (United Kingdom): Cambridge Press; 1999. p. 1–34.

12. Booth RJ. General husbandry and medical care of sugar gliders. In: Bonagura JD, editor. Kirk's current veterinary therapy XIII. Philadelphia: WB Saunders; 2000. p. 1157–63.

13. Ness RD, Johnson-Delaney CA. Sugar gliders. In: Quesenberry KE, Carpenter JW, editors. Ferrets, rabbits, and rodents clinical medicine and surgery. 3rd edition. St Louis (MO): Elsevier Inc; 2012. p. 393–410.

14. Brust DM. Gastrointestinal diseases of marsupials. J Exot Pet Med 2009;12(2): 197–208.

15. Dierenfeld ES. Feeding behavior and nutrition of the sugar glider (Petaurus breviceps). Vet Clin North Am Exot Anim Pract 2009;12:209–15.

16. Dierenfeld E, Thomas D, Ives R. Comparison of commonly used diets on intake, digestion, growth, and health in captive sugar gliders (Petaurus breviceps). J Exot Pet Med 2006;15:218–24.

17. Gamble KC. Marsupial care and husbandry. Vet Clin North Am Exot Anim Pract 2004;7:283–98.

18. Johnson-Delaney CA. Feeding sugar gliders. Exotic DVM 1998;1(1):4.

19. Smith JA. Macropod nutrition. Vet Clin North Am Exot Anim Pract 2009;12: 197–208.

20. Munn AJ, Dawson TJ. Mechanistic explanations for drought-related mortality of juvenile red kangaroos: implications for population dynamics and modeling. In: Coulson G, Eldridge M, editors. Macropods: the biology of kangaroos, wallabies and rat-kangaroos. Collingwood (Victoria): CSIRO Publishing; 2010. p. 117–26.

21. Walraven E. Handling and emergency care for common marsupial groups. In: Care of Australian wildlife. Sydney (Australia): New Holland Publishers (Australia) Pty Ltd; 1999. p. 62–74.

22. Mazuri Reference Guide. Mazuri/PMI International Company LLC, Brentwood (MO). Available at: www.mazuri.cl/mazuri-diet-reference-guide.pdf; www.mazuri. com. Accessed November 27, 2013.

23. Reliable Protein Products. Available at: http://zoofood.com. Accessed November 27, 2013.

24. Oxbow Pet Products. Available at: www.oxbowanimalhealth.com. Accessed November 28, 2013.

25. Johnson-Delaney CA. What every veterinarian needs to know about Virginia opossums. Exotic DVM 2005;6(6):38–43.

26. Opossum Society of the United States. 2003. Available at: www. opossumsocietyus.org. Accessed November 24, 2013.

27. McRuer DL, Jones KD. Behavioral and nutritional aspects of the Virginian opossum (Didelphis virginiana). Vet Clin North Am Exot Anim Pract 2009;12:217–36.

28. Chan J, Mahaney MC, Kushwaha R, et al. ABCB4 mediates diet-induced hypercholesterolemia in laboratory opossums. J Lipid Res 2010;51:2922–8.

29. VandeBerg JL, Robinson ES. The laboratory opossum (Monodelphis domestica) in laboratory research. ILAR J 1997;38:4–12.

30. Evans KD, Hewett TA, Clayton CJ, et al. Normal organ weights, serum chemistry, hematology, and cecal and nasopharyngeal bacterial cultures in the gray short-

tailed opossum (Monodelphis domestica). J Am Assoc Lab Anim Sci 2010;49(4): 401–6.

31. Nicholas K, Sharp J, Watt A, et al. The tammar wallaby: a model system to examine domain-specific delivery of milk protein bioactives. Semin Cell Dev Biol 2012;23:547–56.

32. Taggart DA, Schultz DJ, Fletcher TP, et al. Cross-fostering and short-term pouch young isolation in macropodoid marsupials: implications for conservation and species management. In: Coulson G, Eldridge M, editors. Macropods, the biology of kangaroos, wallabies and rat-kangaroos. Collingwood (Victoria): CSIRO publishing; 2010. p. 261–78.

33. Johnson-Delaney CA. Reproductive medicine of companion marsupials. Vet Clin North Am Exot Anim Pract 2002;5:537–53.

34. Booth R. Macropods. In: Gage LJ, editor. Hand-rearing wild and domestic animals. Ames (IA): Iowa State Press; 2002. p. 63–74.

35. Barnes M. Sugar gliders. In: Gage LJ, editor. Hand-rearing wild and domestic animals. Ames (IA): Iowa State Press; 2002. p. 55–62.

36. Henness AM. Infant diet (through 4 mo.) 'Possum Tales' (newsletter of the National Opossum Society) 1995;(3–4):5.

37. Taylor P. Opossums. In: Gage LJ, editor. Hand-rearing wild and domestic animals. Ames (IA): Iowa State Press; 2002. p. 45–54.

Ferret Nutrition

Cathy A. Johnson-Delaney, BS, DVM

KEYWORDS

- Nutrition • Ferret • Carnivore • Diet

KEY POINTS

- The domestic ferret is a strict carnivore, requiring high protein and fat levels in the diet.
- The ferret's anatomy and physiology are adapted to its carnivorous diet.
- There are several commercial ferret diets that adequately meet the ferret's nutritional needs.
- Nutritional diseases have been reported in ferrets as seen in other species.
- There are specific nutritional considerations for ferrets with insulinoma or who are geriatric.

INTRODUCTION

The domestic ferret (*Mustela putorious furo*) is a strict carnivore, also referred to as an obligate carnivore.[1–3] Its dentition and gastrointestinal (GI) tract are adapted to a carnivorous diet. Its ancestor, the European polecat (*Mustela putorius*), feeds on birds and other small vertebrates. Domesticated ferrets have been fed mink feeds, cat foods, and now mostly subsist on commercial ferret diets formulated specifically to meet their needs.

ANATOMY AND PHYSIOLOGY

As obligate carnivores, ferrets have a very short intestinal tract and lack a cecum and ileocolic valve.[1,3] The gut is essentially a simple tube from stomach to rectum that allows food to pass through too quickly for efficient absorption.[1] The small intestine is approximately 5 times longer than the ferret's body.[1] For comparison, a cat's small intestine is 8 to 10 times the length of its body.[1] The GI transit time is approximately 3 hours.[2,4] Kits may have a more rapid transit time, as little as 1 hour.[1,4] This rapid intestinal transit time contributes to the inefficiency of absorption. Additionally, concentrations of at least some intestinal brush border enzymes (eg, lactase) are lower

Disclosure: None.
Washington Ferret Rescue and Shelter, Box 1034, 11700 Mukilteo Speedway, Suite 201, Mukilteo, WA 98275, USA
E-mail address: cajddvm@hotmail.com

in ferrets than in other species.[1] Weaning-age kits have less lactase per gram of jejunal mucosa than mature rats. This results in soft stool appearance within an hour when an adult ferret drinks an ounce of milk.[1]

Ferrets are spontaneous secretors of hydrochloric acid. It is natural for them and other closely related mustelids (eg, mink, weasels) to store food and to eat small amounts at frequent intervals rather than gorging every day or two like most carnivores.[1] Pet ferrets often take their kibble and hide it for snacking.

CLINICAL SIGNIFICANCE OF THE FERRET'S GI SYSTEM

Because of the rapid intestinal transit time and small meals eaten, ferrets should not be fasted more than 3 hours before surgery. Four to six hours is generally successful in reducing gut content as much as an overnight fast does for a dog or cat.[1,4] Growing kits or juveniles become irritable and may be likely to bite after a long fast. Ferrets with insulinomas may become severely hypoglycemic if fasted for more than 1 to 2 hours. If it is necessary to empty the GI tract in a ferret with insulinoma, it is acceptable to continue to feed the ferret concentrated, low-volume supplements, such as Nutri-Cal (Vetoquinol USA, Inc, Ft Worth, TX) until 1 to 2 hours before surgery.[1] On ultrasound or radiographic examination if there is food in the stomach after a 4- to 6-hour fast it may indicate delayed emptying or the potential possibility of a trichobezoar.

Another effect of the ferret's gut morphology is an unsophisticated gut flora.[1] The usual anaerobic flora abundant in most mammals is scanty in the ferret, probably in part because of the abbreviated large intestine. The large intestine is only approximately 10 cm long in an adult male.[1] Ferrets raised in an isolator after cesarean derivation had none of the intestinal problems common to other germ-free animals; however, they did require vitamin K supplementation, suggesting that gut flora does play an essential part in some of the digestive processes.[1] Ferrets treated for weeks or months with broad-spectrum antibiotics do not seem to experience GI upsets, such as diarrhea.[1]

DENTITION

The adult dental formula of the ferret is I3/3 C1/1 P3/3 M1/2, which equals 34.[5,6] There is exaggeration of the carnassial teeth (fourth maxillary premolar) and dimunition and shift in function of the molariform teeth for shearing.[5,6] There is a loss of grinding function in the molars, and it is not unusual to find the mandibular second molar has only partial or no occlusion with the maxillary dentition.[5] In many cases it does not come into actual contact with the maxillary first molar.[5] These teeth are located in the back of the jaw where leverage and muscular force is the greatest, likely to serve to crack bones, rather than to grind food.[5] Another adaptation is the overlapping and interdigitation of the mandibular arcade by the maxillary arcade, which prevents lateral movement of the mandibles. This prevents the grinding motions necessary to process plant materials and abrasive foods, but does allow for the dorsoventral movement necessary for the cheek teeth and carnassials to shear tissue-based foods.[5] The temporomandibular joint effectively locks the mandible into the skull preventing the loss of bite force during predation.[5] The maxillary canines and cheek teeth are aligned into what effectively become arches, which is a common adaptation of carnivores that strengthens the skull without adding bone mass.[5] The canine teeth form a tight interlock when the mouth is closed.[6] The biomechanics of these adaptations are markedly different from those of herbivores. It is likely that the shift from a whole-prey diet to one of dry kibble may have deleterious impact on the function of the ferret's specific dental adaptations, although this has yet to be the focus of a published research study.[5]

Kibble is crunchy and abrasive, a selling point to reduce dental calculus, but chewing kibble may cause structural changes to the tooth and underlying boney support.[5] This ultimately causes excessive wear of the tooth and may result in fractures or loss of the tooth. In short, the ferret's dentition is not well-suited to having to grind kibble.

COMMERCIAL DIETS

Years ago ranched ferrets were fed a mink diet. But pet ferrets do not like the fish flavor and instead prefer chicken flavor. Fish-source diets may cause vomiting in some ferrets.[4] A whole-prey diet or a balanced fresh or freeze-dried carnivore diet may be most appropriate and such diets are currently fed in many areas of the world with great success.[2,7] Clean sources of prey food, such as chicks, mice, and rats, are now available in many areas thanks to the reptile market, which uses these foods for carnivorous pets.[2] If an owner does not want to feed a 100% whole-prey or raw diet, consider the occasional treat of a whole mouse or chick as valuable environmental enrichment. The stools of a ferret on a whole-prey diet are very firm and of low volume and odor.[2] Grocery store cat foods are very palatable because of their coating of animal fat, but nutritionally are inadequate for any stage of a ferret's life. Minimally stressed pet ferrets may get by on these foods for years, but nutritional deficiencies are quickly revealed in breeding animals. The acid test of a complete diet is to feed it to a large group of young animals, then allow them to reproduce. Some premium dry cat foods and pelleted ferret diets have proved to meet all the ferret's nutritional requirements for growth and reproduction.[1] The most common type of diet fed to pet ferrets in the United States is in the form of dry kibble. Several brands are available. **Table 1** lists analysis of several commercial diets that meet a ferret's needs for growth and reproduction.

FOOD CONSIDERATIONS

To compensate for the inefficiency of its digestive tract, the ferret requires a concentrated diet that is high in protein and fat and low in fiber.[1] The main source of calories should be fat. When fat is metabolized, it releases twice as much energy as either carbohydrates or protein.[1] Diets with as much as 40% fat have been fed to ferrets without apparent injury, but 15% to 30% fat for pets is generally considered sufficient.[1,2,4]

Unless ferrets are constantly fed high-fat treats, most ferrets eat as much as they want without becoming pathologically obese. They normally increase their food intake by at least 30% in the winter, gaining a great deal of weight by depositing subcutaneous fat.[1] The rule of thumb is that an adult ferret eats about 43 g/kg body weight of dry food per day. The ferret eats up to 10 meals a day if given feed ad libitum.[9] Seasonal obesity is not harmful and should be considered normal. As the hours of daylight increase in the spring, the ferret reduces its food intake, metabolizes the extra fat, and regains its long, slender shape. If the photoperiod does not vary seasonally, the natural physiologic change may not occur. Some ferrets may remain either lean or plump all the time.[1] A study looking at the dietary preferences and digestion of commercial feline diets in cats and ferrets showed that both preferred diets of higher fat content. However, the ferret differed in its ability to use the cat food, and the conclusion of the study was that ferrets cannot be used as model animals for cats for either preference or digestibility studies![10]

Ferrets require a higher protein level in the diet than most animals, probably because of the inefficiency of their digestive process or for a need for certain amino acids in short supply than to a greater protein requirement at the cellular level.[1] The basic diet for adults should have a crude protein level between 30% and 35% and be composed primarily of high-quality meat sources, not grains. The fat content should be between 15% and 30%.[2] Kits do not thrive on a diet containing less than 30% protein. Conception rate, litter size, and survivability of the kits improve when the protein concentration is increased to 35% to 40% of the breeding ferrets' diet.[1] Protein quality is as important as concentration.[1] The protein in the best-quality animal

Table 1
Analysis of commercial diets that support growth and reproduction

	Diet A	Diet B	Diet C	Diet D
Nutrient				
Crude protein %	39.8	39.0	38.0	36.5
Crude fat %	20.2	20.5	20.0	23.3
Crude fiber %	2.2	2.6	4.0	1.4
Moisture %	4.2	10.0	12.0	7.5
Ash %	7.4	6.5	7.5	6.5
Carbohydrate %	26.2	21.4	17.5	24.8
Amino acid profile				
Arginine %	2.52	2.05	2.5	2.4
Cystine %	0.45	0.59	0.56	0.44
Histidine %	0.91	0.61	0.75	0.95
Isoleucine %	1.67	1.44	1.40	1.30
Leucine %	3.09	3.20	2.60	2.55
Lysine %	2.74	2.02	2.20	2.40
Methionine %	1.18	0.85	0.80	1.05
Phenylalanine %	1.64	1.48	1.30	1.40
Tyrosine %	1.32	0.76	1.20	1.10
Threonine %	1.90	1.31	1.40	1.50
Tryptophan %	0.33	0.29	0.32	0.38
Valine %	1.99	1.77	1.70	1.72
Taurine %	0.25	0.24	0.52	0.24
Fat				
Linoleic acid %	3.0	2.76	3.0	4.50
Minerals				
Calcium %	1.2	1.4	1.4	1.28
Phosphorus %	1.05	1.25	1.30	0.88
Ca/P ratio	1.14:1	1.12:1	1.08:1	1.45:1
Potassium %	0.75	0.56	0.70	0.68
Magnesium %	0.10	0.12	0.10	0.09
Sodium %	0.55	0.40	0.40	0.42
Iron ppm (mg/kg)	360	320	305	240
Copper mg/kg	30	24	22	24
Manganese mg/kg	70	72	75	80
Zinc mg/kg	145	232	235	240
Iodine mg/kg	2.6	2.0	1.9	2.0
Selenium mg/kg	0.3	0.6	0.2	0.35

(continued on next page)

	Diet A	Diet B	Diet C	Diet D
Table 1 *(continued)*				
Vitamins				
A (IU/kg)	35,100	25,100	31,765	25,000
D₃ (IU/kg)	2200	3700	3560	1800
E (IU/kg)	155	250	235	300
K (ppm, mg/kg)	1.2	3.2	3.0	2.0
Thiamin mg/kg	12.8	56	54	45
Riboflavin mg/kg	25	20	22	55
Niacin mg/kg	95	110	128	120
Pantothenic acid mg/kg	25	26.2	25	35
Folic acid mg/kg	1.5	4.3	4.4	3.0
Pyridoxine mg/kg	12.5	17.5	28	35
Biotin mg/kg	0.60	0.48	0.43	10.2
Metabolizable energy kcal/g	3.89	4.0	4.2	4.35

Diet A: Marshall Premium Ferret (Marshall Pet Products, North Rose, NY, www.marshallpet.com).
Diet B: Purina High Density Ferret Lab Diet 5L14 (Lab Diet, St Louis, MO, www.labdiet.com).
Diet C: Mazuri Ferret (PMI Nutrition International LLC, Brentwood, MO, www.mazuri.com/product_pdfs/5M08.pdf).
Diet D: Totally Ferret Active Show & Pet Formula (Performance Foods, Inc, Broomfield, CO).
Data from Refs.[1,7,8]

feeds is 85% to 90% digestible as compared with less than 75% in many grocery store cat foods.[1] A food with 30% crude protein of 70% digestibility really only contains 21% available protein, and may be mainly cereals.[1] The diet of an obligate carnivore like a cat or ferret must contain predominantly animal protein and fat. Infectious and metabolic diseases are prevalent in growing, gestating, or lactating ferrets when grains are the major source of protein.[1]

The proportion of carbohydrate is higher in a grain-based diet than in a meat-based diet. Grains are used to help the pellet hold its shape. Very high levels of plant proteins in the diet can lead to urolithiasis.[2,11] The hardness of the kibble may promote excessive dental wear and disease.[2,5] The only natural source of carbohydrates for mustelids is the gut content of their prey.[1] Dogs make good use of carbohydrates as an energy source in diets containing more than 60% carbohydrates. Cats, however, with a shorter intestinal tract and different metabolism, do poorly if carbohydrates exceed 40% of the diet.[1] Ferrets have an even shorter intestinal tract, comparatively deficient in brush-border enzymes, and are less able than cats to absorb enough calories from carbohydrates.[1,12] The simple gut flora and rapid passage time through the colon does not allow a ferret to make as much use of complex carbohydrates as other species.[1,12] The nitrogen-free extract in a chemical food analysis is made up of soluble, digestible carbohydrates (eg, sugar or starch). Insoluble carbohydrates are referred to as fiber. The digestibility of soluble complex carbohydrates is improved by cooking. However, fiber remains completely indigestible by simple-stomached animals. Fiber attracts fluid to the lumen of the gut, increasing stool volume and having a beneficial effect when natural laxative is required. "Lite" pet foods designed for weight reduction are based on the principle of feeding a high-fiber food of low digestibility to allow the animal to lose weight without always feeling hungry.[1] Increasing dietary fiber causes the volume of stool to increase in ferrets as it does in dogs and cats, but it also induces a relative protein-calorie deficiency in the ferret.[1] Ferrets cannot eat enough low-density food to meet their maintenance requirements.[1] Simply, the ferret has little ability to digest fiber.[13] Pet ferrets sometimes develop a taste for high-carbohydrate or high-fiber foods, such as fruits or vegetables, but they derive little nutritional benefit from them.[1] Treat foods consisting of cereals are likewise not digestible, but may be extremely palatable because they are sugar-coated.[2] A study looking at sweet receptor gene (Tas1r2) and preference for sweet stimuli in species of carnivore has found that ferrets preferred fructose over other sugars. Ferrets did not respond to artificial sweeteners. They have an intact Tas1r2 gene.[14]

SPECIFIC NUTRITIONAL REQUIREMENTS

Although the exact nutritional requirements of ferrets have not been determined by feeding trials with defined diets as have been done for other animals, diets that have sustained reproduction and growth of generations of healthy kits must meet or exceed their minimum requirements.[1] Daily metabolizable energy intakes for ferrets have been estimated to range from 200 to 300 calories (kcals) per kilogram body weight. Energy intakes above maintenance are needed for growth, gestation, and lactation.[3,4] **Table 2** lists energy needs of ferrets in kilocalorie metabolizable energy per day with increases needed for differing calorie requirements. Examples of the nutritional content of several complete rations that support growth, gestation, and lactation are shown in **Table 1**. These diets contain 3.9 to 4.58 kcal of metabolizable energy per gram of food.[1] Other premium cat foods, ferret foods, or mink foods of similar analysis and quality of ingredients may be expected to provide adequate nutrition for a breeding ferret and more than adequate nutrition for a pet.[1] Palatability is a major concern when considering the benefits of any food for a ferret. For example, a well-balanced mink diet with a strong fishy flavor may be so unpalatable that pets steadfastly refuse to eat it.[1] **Table 3** lists nutrients provided by some of the ingredients found in the ferret diets.

Table 2
Energy needs of ferrets (kcal ME/day) increase above maintenance for growth, reproduction, and lactation

Body Weight (g)	Multiples of Maintenance[a] (kcal ME/d)				
	1	1.5	2.0	2.5	3.0
600	150	225	300	375	450
700	175	262	350	438	525
800	200	300	400	500	600
900	225	338	450	562	675
1000	250	375	500	625	750
1200	300	450	600	750	900
1400	350	525	700	875	1050
1600	400	600	800	1000	1200
1800	450	675	900	1125	1350
2000	500	750	1000	1250	1500
2200	550	825	1100	1375	1650

Abbreviation: ME, metabolizable energy.
[a] Maintenance is defined as the daily ME intake (kcal/day) of healthy adults in comfortable surroundings (250 [W]), in which W = body weight in kg.
Data from Kupersmith DS. A practical overview of small mammal nutrition. Sem Avian Exotic Pet Med 1998;7(3):141–7.

Table 3
Nutrients provided by some ingredients of ferret diets and supplements

Ingredient or Supplement	Crude Protein (%)	Fat (%)	Fiber (%)	Carbohydrate (%)	Calories per gram	Moisture (%)	Calcium/ Phosphorus Ratio
Poultry by-product	58.7	13.1	2.3	3.6	2.8	7	1.9:1
Ground beef	20.7	10.0	Not listed	3.5 calculated	1.8	68.3	1:19
Fresh liver (beef)	19.9	3.8	0.1	6.5	1.4	69.7	1:35
Liver meal	71.4	17.0	1.5	3.4	Not listed	8	1:2
Wheat	14.2	1.8	2.6	68.7	Not listed	89	1:10.5
Rice	7.9	1.7	8.9	65.6	Not listed	89	1:4.7
Soybean meal	42.9	4.8	5.9	30.4	Not listed	90	1:2.3
Corn	10.9	4.3	2.9	80.4	NL	11	1:1
Nutri-Cal 1 tsp (6 g)	0.04 g	2.1 g	0.22 g	2.8 g	26.5	14	6:1
Ferrettone 1 mL	0	0.9	0	0	8.7	Not listed	Not listed
Whole cooked egg (1 egg, 50 g)	6.45	5.8	Not listed	Not listed	82	73.7	1:4
Whole milk (3.5% fat, 10 mL)	0.35	0.35	0	0.56	6.5	87.4	Not listed
Raisins (6 small or 3 large yellow; 3 g)	0.1 g	0.02 g	0.2 g	2.4 g	9.5	Not listed	Not listed
Cheerios (10–11 pieces; 1 g)	0.5 g	0.2 g	0.2 g	2.1 g	11.9	Not listed	Not listed
Baby food chicken 10 mL	1.3 g	0.68 g	0	0	11	80	Not listed
Science Diet A/D 10 mL	1.1 g	0.7 g	0.03 g	0.4 g	12	77	1:1

Data from Bell JA. Ferret nutrition. Vet Clin North Am Exot Anim Pract 1999;2(1):169–92.

Examples of diets that failed to meet the nutritional requirements of breeding ferrets are shown in **Table 4**. These diets have a higher carbohydrate content and lower protein content than those in **Table 1**. Furthermore, the protein was a lower quality, a fact that cannot be appreciated from either the analysis or the ingredients list, but which made a significant difference to the animals.[1] Low-quality meat or poultry meal contains too much indigestible protein (eg, feathers or hooves), too much bone, and too little muscle meat. The result is a diet deficient in essential amino acids. The serious consequences of feeding poor-quality meat protein or too high a proportion of cereal protein to breeding ferrets include but are not limited to urinary tract, GI, and respiratory infections; urolithiasis; reproductive failure; and poor growth of kits.[1]

Although little research has been done on the requirements of ferrets, a great deal of effort has been put into developing diets for ranch mink by feeding analyzed diets to breeding mink and observing the results.[1] Although this does provide an insight into the minimum requirements of minks and ferrets, the information is not complete because the interactions of individual nutrients are uncontrolled in these studies.[1] Before the true requirements of ferrets can be known, purified diets must be tested on large groups of animals, so that a single nutrient may be varied and its effect analyzed independent of other variables. There are many gaps in what is known about ferrets' specific requirements.[1] For example, arginine and methionine are limiting amino acids in the diets of other animals, and probably of ferrets, but their actual requirements in ferrets are unknown.[1] An animal eats enough food to meet its requirements for the limiting amino acids, even if that means consuming two or three times more than the requirement amount of other amino acids.[1] The excess is metabolized and used for energy, and the nitrogen is excreted by the kidneys. The high blood urea nitrogen of healthy ferrets suggests that they usually have an excess of protein, but their physical condition suffers when the diet contains less than 30% protein. Providing all of the limiting amino acids in the required concentrations in a lower protein diet should make it possible to maintain the ferret in the same state of good health and productivity that presently necessitates that their diet contain 35% crude protein.[1]

Taurine deficiency has been linked with dilated cardiomyopathy and retinal degeneration in cats. Although dilated cardiomyopathy and retinal degeneration are found

Table 4
Guaranteed analysis of two diets associated with urolithiasis and poor reproductive performance in ferrets

Analysis (%)	Diet #1	Diet #2
Crude protein	31.0	30.0
Crude fat	16.0	8.0
Fiber	3.0	4.5
Ash	8.0	6.3
Moisture	11.0	12.0
Carbohydrate	31.0	39.2
First 8 listed ingredients	Poultry by-product meal, ground wheat, ground yellow corn, soybean meal, wheat germ meal, animal fat preserved with BHA, meat and bone meal, salt	Whole kernel corn, soybean meal, corn gluten meal, poultry by-product meal, whole wheat, animal fat preserved with mixed tocopherols (source of vitamin E), brewers rice, fish meal

Data from Bell JA. Ferret nutrition. Vet Clin North Am Exot Anim Pract 1999;2(1):169–92.

in the ferrets, there is no hard evidence that taurine deficiency causes either one.[1] However, it is recommended that taurine be added to ferret diets at the same level as is present in premium cat foods.[1] The author has used taurine supplementation in ferrets with dilated cardiomyopathy and has clinically seen improvement in the condition. It is also assumed that arachidonic acid is an essential fatty acid for ferrets as it is for cats, because it is present only in animal tissues. Fish oil is a good source of arachidonic acid, and hence the beautiful pelts grown by fitch ferrets that eat pelleted mink food. Meat-based diets usually are not deficient in either taurine or arachidonic acid.[1]

MINERALS AND VITAMINS

Although very little research has been done to evaluate ferret mineral requirements, mink diets have been extensively researched, and their requirements seem to be similar to those of other animals including cats.[1] It is safe to assume that ferrets have similar requirements. The calcium-phosphorus ratio should be at least 1:1. Commercial formulations generally contain ratios 1.2:1 to 1.7:1.[15] The diets listed in **Table 1** show the varying ratios and because all minerals have proved adequate for growing and lactating ferrets, the amount of each mineral in the food must meet or exceed their requirements.[1] Milk and meat meal that includes bone are well-balanced sources of calcium and phosphorus, but muscle meat or liver and grains are low in calcium.[1] A diet of meat alone induces a calcium deficiency and gross skeletal abnormalities.[1] Signs of calcium or calcium deficiency include tooth loss, skeletal deformities in kits, and spontaneous fractures. Ferrets on high-quality cat or ferret foods do not have mineral deficiencies unless they are persistently fed a supplement of a medication (eg, tetracycline) that drastically unbalances the diet.[1] Commercial diets are considered adequate in iron, copper, sodium, chlorine, zinc, magnesium, iodine, and potassium.[15] Other microminerals called trace elements in addition to the above include cobalt, chromium, and molybdenum, and are usually combined with other nutrients and never added to the diet in pure form. Additionally, fluoride, nickel, vanadium, silicon, and tin are necessary but in minute and organic form in the diet.[7]

Oversupplementation of vitamin A in liver or concentrated nutritional products induces skeletal abnormalities in cats and has occurred in ferrets fed a diet of raw liver exclusively.[1] Vitamin E is added to high-quality pet foods as an antioxidant. Ferrets fed extra fat (eg, linoleic acid) might require more vitamin E, but deficiencies are unlikely to occur in pets fed pelleted diets.[1] Vitamin E deficiency was a problem when ferrets were fed raw meat or fish that contained rancid fat. Steatitis has been seen in young ferrets fed diets containing an excessive amount of fish or horsemeat.[13] The ferret foods listed in **Table 1** probably all contain an excess of vitamin E for normal animals.[1] Other information on vitamin requirements of ferrets have been determined because of their use as laboratory research animals. Ferrets unlike cats are able to convert betacarotene to vitamin A, and in the diet this conversion is stimulated by 1% taurocholate (cholic acid conjugated with taurine), 23% fat, 40% protein, and alpha-tocopherol (vitamin E) at physiologic doses.[1,16] However, ferrets convert betacarotene to vitamin A inefficiently, and the diet should contain added vitamin A.[15,17] Studies also have been done showing that ferrets had a higher body weight gain when supplemented with betacarotene.[18] The natural source of vitamin E for a carnivorous animal is the liver of its prey.[1] Studies have been done using the ferret as a model for lung cancer, and have found that the addition of betacarotene, alpha-tocopherol (vitamin E), and ascorbic acid (vitamin C) effectively blocked the formation of preneoplastic lung lesions and lung cancer tumor formation.[19,20] Another interesting study looked at tobacco smoke induction of changes in the gastric mucosa of ferrets as a model for gastric cancer and found that lycopene effectively prevented the damage.[21] In the author's opinion, this may have implications for its use in consideration of gastric health.

Vitamin D requirements may depend on dietary concentrations of calcium and phosphorus or on the duration of exposure to UV-B light.[15] Other factors include dietary calcium to phosphorus ratio, physiologic state of development, and gender. Rachitic changes and abnormal bone development may occur when the diet is deficient in vitamin D, calcium, or phosphorus especially when exposure to ultraviolet light is minimized.[15] Commercial ferret diets generally have sufficient vitamin D, calcium, and phosphorus in the appropriate ratios. Most pet ferrets receive little to no UV-B light.

Vitamin K metabolic need has not been established in the ferret, but it is likely that a dry diet concentration of 1.0 mg menadione/kg would sustain normal plasma prothrombin levels.[15] A deficiency may result in hypoprothrombinemia and hemorrhage. Vitamin K toxicity has been linked with kernicterus and hemolytic anemia in other species.[15]

The thiamin concentration in commercially available ferret diets is generally considered adequate. A diet of raw eggs may predispose ferrets to thiamin deficiency.[15] Thiamine deficiency disease has been reported on ferret farms in New Zealand that fed a diet consisting of fish containing thiaminase.[15] It was seen in weanling growing and adult ferrets. It was characterized by anorexia, lethargy, marked dyspnea, prostration, and convulsions.[7,15] Signs disappeared after parenteral injections of vitamin B complex (5 mg daily for 3 days).[15] Death caused by depression of the respiratory center may occur with toxic doses, likely in excess of 200 mg/kg body weight.[15]

Riboflavin needs are considered met with less than 3 mg/kg. Commercial ferret diets contain in excess of this amount.[15] Acute deficiency may result in decreased respiratory rate, hypothermia, weakness, and coma. Chronic deficiency may result in anorexia, muscular weakness, dermatitis, microcytic-hypochromic anemia, corneal vascularization-opacification, and reduced erythrocyte and urine riboflavin concentration.[15]

A sufficient amount of pyridoxin is considered to be 1 mg of vitamin B_6 per kilogram dry matter. Commercial ferret diets contain eight times this level. Deficiency in mink showed testicular atrophy, aspermia, and degeneration. Absorption sterility occurs in females.[15]

Vitamin B_{12} deficiency has not been described in the ferret.[15] Commercial diet amounts are considered adequate. Vitamin B_{12} deficiency has been linked with macrocytic hypochromic, macrocytic normochromic, normocytic hypochromic, or normocytic normochromic anemias in other species.[15]

Folic acid synthesis by intestinal bacteria has not been studied in the ferret, but commercial diets are considered to have adequate amounts that bacterial synthesis is not needed.[15] In mink, folic acid at 0.5 mg/kg of dry feed causes a remission of such symptoms as erratic appetite, poor weight gain, glossitis, leucopenia, and hypochromic anemia.[15]

Biotin is provided in commercial diets upward of 200 μg biotin per kilogram dry matter leading to 10 μg/kg body weight daily.[15] This level is approximately twice the level required for optimal growth in dogs.[15] Deficiency may result in alopecia, hyperkeratosis, graying of fur, conjunctivitis, and fatty liver.[7,15]

Niacin must be supplied although the metabolic conversion of tryptophan to niacin and has not been systematically studied in the ferret.[15] Mink cannot metabolize enough to meet requirements.[15] Commercial ferret diets provide several times the 20 mg/kg dry diet that is stated as a requirement for mink.[15] Deficiency has been linked with anorexia, profuse salivation, diarrhea, GI inflammation, hemorrhagic necrosis, dehydration, and emaciation in other species. High doses have been linked with vasodilation, pruritus, and cutaneous desquamation in other species.[15]

Pantothenic acid requirements are probably about 500 to 750 μg/kg body weight based on the absence of deficiency signs in ferrets consuming a commercial ferret diet.[15] Deficiency in the ferret may result in poor appetite, slow growth, reduced blood cholesterol and total lipid levels, loss of conditioned reflexes, alopecia, vomiting, intermittent diarrhea, GI disorders, convulsions, and coma.[15]

Choline requirements link with dietary concentration of methionine. Both choline and methionine may serve as methyl donors in metabolism, with the dietary supply of one tending to spare the need for the other. The interaction of these has not been systematically studied in ferrets.[15] Deficiency has led to elevated plasma phosphatase activity and blood prothrombin times. Toxicity may cause an increased alkalination of urine and decreased ammonia excretion.[15]

WATER

Ferrets require approximately three times as much water as dry matter food and should have fresh drinking water constantly available. They prefer to drink from a dish rather than a dropper bottle, and should be given this opportunity at least once daily ensuring that their consumption of dry pellets is not limited by their water intake. Heavy crocks are the best water containers, because most ferrets rest their front feet on the edge of a dish as they drink, and may tip over a lighter container.[1] Many pet ferrets also like to play in water making a water crock problematic.

SELECTING A COMPLETE DIET FOR A PET FERRET

Most pet ferrets are acquired either as kits or young juveniles from pet shops or from private breeders, or they are acquired as older juveniles or adults from shelters. A pet may come to its new owner with strongly established preferences for flavors and food textures. Once they have been accustomed to a diet, ferrets expect to find that food and no other in their dish every day. New owners must be educated on the basics of ferret nutrition and urge them to continue with the balanced diet the ferret is already used to. People buying a kit from a pet store may remain completely unaware of the animal's requirements depending on what the pet shop personnel tells them. A pet shop employee may suggest an expensive premium cat food rather than the ferret food currently being fed the kit. The owner may decide that he or she can get by with a cheaper cat food from the grocery store, leading to malnourishment of the ferret. Most kits readily accept cat food because of its high palatability, even though nutritionally it is not acceptable. Even after selecting a good base diet, many ferret owners decide to give their ferret a taste of their own favorite foods. Ferrets end up snacking on bananas, raisins, apples, ice cream, potato chips, coffee creamer, carbonated drinks, beer, pizza, cereal, and so forth. Ferrets are utterly self-indulgent and gorge themselves on anything they take a liking to. Left to themselves, they eat only their favorite foods, eventually becoming grossly malnourished.[1] Veterinarians who examine a pet shop ferret soon after purchase should advise the owner to select the ferret's diet carefully and limit snack foods that will unbalance the diet.[1]

MAINTENANCE DIETS

A pet ferret's maintenance diet should be 30% to 35% crude protein and 15% to 30% fat.[1,2,9,13] Meat or poultry, meat or poultry meals, or their by-products should appear first in the list of ingredients and preferably several more times in the ingredients list.[1] Other animal products, such as liver and eggs, are included in the highest-quality foods. Although ferret diets, such as Totally Ferret (Performance Foods, Inc, Broomfield, CO) and Marshall Premium Ferret Diet (Marshall Pet Products, North Rose, NY) were formulated for ferrets from babyhood to old age, some premium cat foods have also proved satisfactory. Although the most expensive commercial diet is not necessarily best for any individual ferret, the cheapest ones are certainly the worst.[1] Ferrets fed dog food eventually die, either directly of malnutrition or of GI or respiratory infections arising from poor immune function.[1]

UNSUITABLE DIETS

Grocery store and generic cat foods are incomplete diets. Serious health problems have been directly or indirectly related to feeding a base diet of low-cost grocery store or generic cat food to ferrets. The list of ingredients for these foods usually starts with ground yellow corn. Metabolism of cereal proteins alkalinizes the animal's urine, encouraging struvite urolith formation in ferrets and cats.[1,15] The normal pH of the urine should be less than 6.5.[11] When diets high in cereal proteins are fed to pregnant or lactating jills, 5% to 10% have uroliths, and a significant number require emergency surgery to remove large single or smaller multiple struvite uroliths.[1,11] Not only is the protein in grocery store cat foods predominantly from cereals, there is too little of it for ferrets, and the proportion that comes from meat is usually of poor quality. Supplementing the ferret with the right balance of whole cooked egg, milk, and minced ground meat or liver corrects the amino acid deficiencies caused by a steady diet of generic cat food. However, fat must also be added, because generic cat foods contain only 8% to 10% fat, which is approximately half of what ferrets require, and a high proportion of carbohydrate.[1]

Young ferrets on protein-deficient diets grow poorly, and immune dysfunction makes them more susceptible to respiratory and GI infections.[1] This is particularly noticeable in groups of pet shop kits that do very well despite multiple stressors as long as they are well nourished. When poor nutrition is superimposed on stress and exposure to pathogens, they develop respiratory infections, clinical coccidiosis, and heavy flea and ear mite infestations. Juveniles raised on low-quality cat food are more likely to develop clinical *Helicobacter* gastritis and ulcers and proliferative colitis.[1]

Nutritional steatitis has been described in ferrets fed a high level of dietary polyunsaturated fat (PUFA).[7,15] In all species reported with this disease it has been caused by feeding a diet high in PUFA and/or deficient in vitamin E. Mink are particularly sensitive.[15] A dietary supplement of 75 to 150 mg/ferret/day of vitamin E is advised when feeding ferrets a high-PUFA diet.[15] This is similar to the mink. The high level of selenium found in the liver of ferrets with steatitis did not reduce the toxicity of the high-PUFA content of the feed, although selenium does protect tissue against lipoperioxidases.[15]

Osteodystrophia fibrosa (nutritional hyperparathyroidism) mainly caused by feeding an all-meat diet with no calcium supplementation has been documented in ferrets.[7,15] True rickets (hypophosphorosis and/or hypovitaminosis D) has not been reported in ferrets. All ages are susceptible, but rapid growth predisposes ferrets to the disease if the diet is inadequate in calcium, phosphorus, and vitamin D.[15] Affected ferrets are reluctant to move, cannot support their own weight, and the typical posture is abduction of the forelegs. The bones are soft, pliable, and fractures may be present.[15] This has been diagnosed predominantly in instances where a commercial ferret diet is not being fed. On necropsy, the bones are osteoporotic with typical lesions of osteodystrophia fibrosa. The parathyroid glands are hyperplastic.[15]

Zinc toxicity has been reported in ferrets exposed to excessive levels of zinc in the diet that were leached from galvanized feeding pans and water dishes.[15] All ages are susceptible. Affected animals have pale mucous membranes caused by anemia. Posterior weakness and lethargy was seen. This problem was reported on two ferret farms in New Zealand.[15]

Salt poisoning was caused by feeding a diet of 100% salted fish. Clinical signs are typical of those seen in other species, particularly pigs, affected with the disease.[15] Animals are significantly depressed and have periodic choriform spasms, seen 24 to 96 hours after ingestion of excessive salty diets. Death ensures shortly thereafter.[15] Pathology is restricted to the brain, which is edematous and shows coning of the cerebellum.[15] Nonsuppurative eosinophilic meningitis was also found.[15]

SWITCHING TO AN OPTIMAL DIET

A young ferret accustomed to a mixture of several premium cat or ferret foods is usually easy to keep on feeding just one brand of ferret food. Young ferrets imprint on food by smell at a very young age, and develop strong food preferences by the time they are a few months old. Therefore, regardless of the diet strategy that is chosen, ferrets should be exposed to a variety of food tastes, textures, smalls, and different protein sources as juveniles so their diet has more flexibility as an adult. This can be extremely helpful when ferrets experience medical conditions that may require altered diets.[2] Older ferrets, however, may be quite stubborn and difficult to switch from that lower-quality "tasty" cat food. Changing an adult ferret's eating habits can be frustrating and stressful for the owner and the ferret.[1] When a complete change is necessary, offer a smorgasbord of high-quality foods mixed with the diet that the ferret is used to. Some ferrets would rather fight than switch foods. They make a clear statement by digging all the new food out of the dish, or deliberately carrying it pellet by pellet into their litter box.[1] A sudden change is risky because some ferrets fast to the point of starvation rather than eat the new food. Instead of giving up and allowing the pet to eat the generic kibble that it craves, feed it palatable, balanced supplements, such as Nutri-Cal mixed into a soup of ground pellets (mix food it is used to plus the diet you are trying to get it to convert to so that the new tastes are part of the powder), plus mix in some baby food chicken or turkey creating "Dook Soup" (**Box 1**, **Table 5**). Gradually decrease the water content of the Dook Soup and increase the proportion of the correct diet in the ground powder until the ferret is converted (**Fig. 1**). Unfortunately, using soup for conversion also is fraught with problems. Some ferrets decide that they would rather eat soup than kibble at all and will not switch back to kibble. Have kibble available always and make the soup more and more thick, and offer it only once or twice daily. Usually a healthy ferret starts back eating kibble, particularly if housed with more than one other ferret that has also been converted to a different kibble. The ferret's weight should be checked at least every other day during conversion. If there is weight loss, go to more frequent feedings of Dook Soup and increase the proportion of the good-quality food ground into the powder used as the basis for the soup.

HIGH-FAT SUPPLEMENTS

A ferret on a good balanced diet, usually kibble, needs no supplementation. Feeding coat conditioners that contain linoleic and other fatty acids adds 9 kcal/g of

> **Box 1**
> **My Dook Soup recipe**
>
> Approximately one meal.
>
> Pulverize/grind regular ferret food into a powder. 1 teaspooon of this plus enough water or chicken broth to make it fluid; it may need to soak for over an hour until it is lumpy chowder consistency. Add 1 teaspoon of this to the Dook Soup.
>
> 1 heaping teaspoon Carnivore Care or Emeraid Exotic Carnivore plus enough water to make a soupy consistency.
>
> 1 teaspoon Nutri-Cal.
>
> 1 teaspoon baby food chicken or turkey, or cooked chicken puree.
>
> Add any additional nutrients, such as powdered taurine 25 to 50 mg as indicated.
>
> Mix all the above ingredients with enough additional chicken broth or water to make it the consistency of split pea soup or whatever the ferret will take off a syringe, spoon, or just lap up.
>
> The ferret may need encouragement to eat. Often you can get him/her started by feeding off a finger or spoon.
>
> Meal: usually 30 mL of soup per 1 kg ferret at least 3 times a day. Need to feed enough to maintain or increase body weight.

metabolized fat, causing the ferret to reduce its intake of the balanced diet.[1] If only a few drops a day are fed as a treat, no harm is done. The most common product used is Ferretone (8-in-1, Spectrum Brands, Inc, Islandia, NY, www.eightinonepet.com). This product does not contain any carbohydrates, unlike other commonly used supplements (Ferretvite; 8-in-1, Spectrum Brands) and Nutri-Cal. As an example of the problems this can cause if a teaspoon (5 mL) of Ferretone is given to a 700-g jill daily, she will reduce her intake by the approximately 40 kcal she acquires in the supplement, which is 20% of her caloric requirement per day. If she is on a good-quality ferret food, this added fat will likely only cause her to gain weight and have a thick coat.[1] If she is on a marginal diet, the added fat will detract from the protein content and

Table 5
Commercial products used in Dook Soup

Nutrient	Emeraid Exotic Carnivore	Carnivore Care	Nutri-Cal
Crude protein (min) %	37.80	45.00	0.68
Crude fat (min) %	34.00	32.00	28.14
Crude fiber (max) %	4.50	3.00	Not listed
Omega 3 fatty acids (min) %	1.40	1.00	Not listed
Omega 6 fatty acids (min) %	11.00	7.60	Not listed
Calcium (min) %	1.00	1.40 (max 1.80)	0.0026
Phosphorus (min) %	0.67	1.20	0.0003
Moisture (max) %	9.00	10.00	14.21
Calories	Calculated, dry weight 5.14 kcal/g	6 kcal/g; 24 kcal/tablespoon	60 kcal/tablespoon

Analysis as listed on the package: Emeraid (Lafeber Company, Cornell, IL); Carnivore Care (Oxbow Animal Health, Murdock, NE); Nutri-Cal (Vetoquinol USA, Inc, Fort Worth, TX).

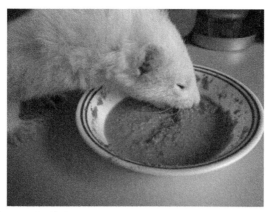

Fig. 1. Ferret eating my Dook Soup.

eventually lead to deficiencies of vitamins and minerals. This ferret will have a poor coat and be in poor condition until the supplementation is ceased.[1] For example, a 700-g jill requires approximately 200 kcal/day and will eat to her caloric requirement. Using a diet that contains 30% crude protein, 8% crude fat, and 4.5% fiber (a typical cat food), which contains approximately 3.5 kcal of metabolizable energy per gram, if it is supplemented with 5 mL of Ferretone every day the ferret will reduce her intake of the dry diet by approximately 40 kcal or 11 g. She was probably consuming approximately 60 g of that diet (18 g of protein), and now she is eating approximately 50 g, which is 15 g of protein. The jill's diet now contains approximately 27% protein, which is primarily from cereal grains and thus is less than 75% digestible. This ferret will have a poor coat, will be thin and abnormally susceptible to infectious diseases, and may even develop struvite urolithiasis.[1]

HIGH-CARBOHYDRATE SUPPLEMENTS

High-carbohydrate supplements (treats) include carbonated drinks, cookies, candy, and raisins. Ferrets love raisins, which are very high in sugar and low in protein and fat. A few raisins a day for a normal ferret on an excellent diet does not cause a nutritional problem, but may pass largely through the intestinal tract with little digestion. In some ferrets they may irritate the GI tract. A ferret on a generic cat food fed a handful of raisins per day raises the carbohydrate intake enough to reduce the consumption of the dry food, inducing protein and fat deficiencies. High-carbohydrate supplements are not needed to augment a ferret's diet.

ACCEPTABLE SUPPLEMENTS (TREATS)

Supplements (treats) should be limited to no more than 10% of the daily caloric intake. A few raisins (9 kcal/teaspoon) or 1 mL of Ferretone (9 kcal/mL) daily does not harm ferrets on good-quality ferret diets.[1] Soft-moist meat or liver snacks manufactured for cats or ferrets make good treats: they contain 50% to 60% moisture and are balanced approximately like a good ferret diet. Check the label for the nutritional content and convert it to a dry matter basis.[1] Other acceptable snacks are a few teaspoonfuls of a high-protein, high-calorie human supplements; baby meats that contain no carbohydrates; egg yolk or whole cooked egg; or small amounts of raw meat or liver (**Fig. 2**). Pureed raw liver or hamburger mixed with egg yolk and milk looks and

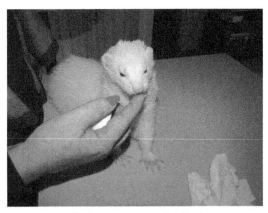

Fig. 2. Ferret licking Nutri-Cal off a finger to start the feeding process.

smells disgusting to people and older ferrets raised on refined, pelleted kibble, but it is universally appealing to kits and contains amino and fatty acids that immediately correct the deficiencies of inadequate diets. Ferrets with sparse coats caused by nutritional deficiencies start growing hair within days. Although some raw meat may contain bacteria or parasites harmful to humans, ferrets and other predators seem very resistant to such infections.[1]

PHYSIOLOGIC STATES THAT REQUIRE SPECIAL NUTRITION
Growth

Weaned kits require an excellent diet if they are to grow to their adult weight. Well-nourished male kits double their weight between 4 (150 g) and 6 weeks of age (300 g) and double it again before they are 9 weeks old (700 g).[1] When fed generic cat foods exclusively, they have poor haircoats, distended abdomens, and a greater susceptibility to respiratory and digestive diseases than kits on high-quality ferret diets. This might not be noticeable to someone who has never seen well-nourished kits, but if weight and health records and photographs are compared, there are dramatic differences in litters on poor- and high-quality diets.[1]

A meat-based dry diet with at least 35% protein and approximately 20% fat should be constantly available to growing kits. A palatable supplement to the dry diet for just-weaned kits is made by mixing the pellets with water and adding cooked eggs and animal fat (or fish oil) to give the resulting porridge the same concentration of protein and calories as the dry diet. Offer the soft food warm once or twice daily. The kits' intake of dry pellets is limited by the availability of drinking water, which should be provided in a heavy crock that needs to be cleaned and refilled at least two to three times a day.[1] A water dropper bottle should also be available. Kits that are placed in the pet stores are usually 6 to 8 weeks old, and are eating a kibble diet, although most stores mix the kibble with water to keep it softened into a mash.

Breeding and Gestation

Jills intended for breeding do not need extra fat, but raising the protein to more than 35% improves conception rate.[1] Jills on poor-quality protein have smaller than average kits and litters. A pregnant jill increases her intake in the last trimester of gestation; because a large litter occupies most of the space in her abdomen, she has to eat frequently. Even a short fast a few days before her due date may induce life-threatening pregnancy toxemia, which is essentially an energy deficit that causes fatty liver syndrome.[1] Extra dishes and water bottles should be provided so that unforeseen accidents do not restrict the jill's intake during the last week of gestation.[1]

Lactating and Weaning

Lactation is heavily dependent on nutrition.[1] A 700-g primiparous jill's litter of 10 kits weighs approximately 80 g at birth and 1000 g 3 to 4 weeks later. Three-week old kits drink a volume of milk replacer (20% fat) equivalent to 30% of their body weight daily, but they probably require less ferret milk, which is perfectly balanced to meet their requirements.[1] After the third week of lactation, the jill daily produces an amount of milk that approaches 40% of her body weight, with a fat content of 10% to 20%.[1] Her caloric requirement doubles if she provides the kits with enough milk to grow normally. Only a constant supply of high-quality food and unrestricted access to water allows this tremendous expenditure of energy. The porridge described for weaned kits should be offered to the nursing jill two to three times daily, first a teaspoonful at a time, and after the litter is 3 weeks old, as much as she will eat.[1] Jills nursing more than 8 kits lose weight no matter what they eat. Allowing the 3-week-old litter access to their mother's soft diet has a sparing effect on her. Even before their eyes open at 30 to 35 days of age, kits are quite able to eat solid food because their deciduous teeth come in at around 2 weeks of age.[2] They may each consume an ounce of food a day when they are only 3 weeks old. The more milk the jill has, the less solid food the kits eat. After their eyes open, they start eating the jill's pellets and any time after 5 weeks may be completely weaned. Litters left with the dam until 6 weeks of age grow faster than early weaned kits.[1]

ILL FERRETS

Any illness that causes anorexia requires nursing care. Anorexic ferrets may develop hepatic lipidosis and hypoglycemia.[22] Usually this means assist-feeding with foods high in protein and fat.[22] Two commercial formulations are available that can be used alone or mixed into Dook Soup to get nutrition into the sick ferret. **Table 5** lists nutrients used in Dook Soup. Emeraid Exotic Carnivore (Lafeber Company, Cornell, IL) is designed to be used alone and can be delivered easily through a gastric tube if the ferret refuses all oral administration (this includes syringing). Carnivore Care (Oxbow Animal Health, Murdock, NE) can also be administered through a gastric tube or by syringe. It can be used solely for the ill ferret. Both powders can be used in combination with ground soaked kibble, baby foods, broth or water, and Nutri-Cal. There are many formulations, but all should maintain the ferret's weight or cause weight gain. The author's preference is to begin by using Emeraid or Carnivore Care alone for the first 24 hours, then to gradually introduce chicken baby food and Nutri-Cal for the next 24 to 48 hours, then gradually mix in the soaked ground regular diet, which thickens up the gruel. It can all be pureed so that it can be administered through a syringe. Most ferrets take syringing or by-hand feeding by dipping a finger in the mix and smearing it on their lips. Many ferrets also take food off a spoon (**Figs. 3** and **4**).

ISLET CELL DISEASE AND DIETARY MANAGEMENT

Insulin-secreting tumors may be benign (insulinomas or β-cell adenomas) or malignant (β-cell carcinomas).[1] Whether histopathologically designated benign or malignant, these tumors secrete insulin and do not differ in their association with clinical signs and shortened life expectancy because of repeated episodes of hypoglycemia.

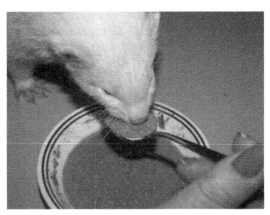

Fig. 3. Ferret eating Dook Soup off a spoon.

Ferrets with islet cell disease present special problems because they are unable to regulate insulin production. Most affected ferrets have multiple pockets of neoplasia that secrete insulin persistently and in response to feeding. Insulin increases tissue uptake of glucose and decreases hepatic gluconeogenesis, effectively lowering blood glucose.[1] The central nervous system depends on blood glucose for normal function. Hypoglycemia causes such signs as lethargy, nausea (shown by pawing at the mouth, hypersalivation, retching), confusion, weakness, convulsions, and eventually coma. Repeated attacks of severe hypoglycemia cause permanent brain damage.[1] The goal of treatment in ferrets with insulin-secreting tumors is to minimize the occurrence of clinical hypoglycemia.

Absorption of glucose stimulates normal and neoplastic β-cells to secrete more insulin and blood glucose may then fall so low that the brain is unable to function normally, and the ferret is found unconscious or convulsing.[1] Even when they appear to be completely unresponsive to other stimuli, hypoglycemic ferrets lick and swallow a glucose solution, 50% dextrose or Nutri-Cal placed on their lips or gums or in the corner of their mouths, and rapidly recover consciousness.[1]

Less severe signs of hypoglycemia are associated with nausea or with weakness and unresponsive behavior.[1] Commonly the ferret seems confused soon after

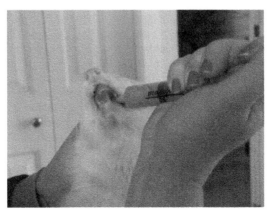

Fig. 4. Syringe feeding using a curved-tip feeding syringe with the tip cut off to allow for more volume to be fed.

awakening or after a few minutes of active play.[1] It either lies flat on its ventrum with eyes appearing glazed or swims, dragging itself along with flipper-like leg movements.[1] Ferrets showing any of these signs recover within a few minutes if given glucose, or 50% dextrose, which immediately raises their blood sugar. However, administration of sugar also stimulates more secretion of insulin and a second episode of hypoglycemia.[1] Administering sugar alone as a treatment of hypoglycemia or as a snack or treat promotes peaks and valleys of blood glucose.[1] Nutri-Cal is a better treatment than a glucose source, such as corn syrup alone, because in addition to sugar it contains fat, which is absorbed and metabolized slowly, maintaining blood glucose at a steady level.[1] Emergency treatment with a sugar source or Nutri-Cal should be followed by a snack of their regular food or Dook Soup.

Ferrets with islet cell disease should have constant access to food and should be encouraged to eat at least every 2 to 4 hours. It is advisable to get them to eat before a play period. The best medical care will not be successful in controlling hypoglycemia unless it is combined with nutritional management.[1] Owners should be advised not to give treats that are high in simple sugars including raisins, peanut butter, and any ferret supplements containing corn syrup or other sugar products.[23] There has been discussion that the ferret should be on a diet high in protein and fats and very low in carbohydrates and fiber, but studies supporting the theory are currently lacking. Further scientific investigations are warranted before specific recommendations can be made.[23] Most commercial ferret diets already fit in this specification.

GERIATRIC FERRETS

Ferrets become geriatric at 3 years of age. As they age, ferrets establish their distinctive habits and food preferences, and changes imposed by humans become progressively more stressful.[12] It is essential to begin feeding a good diet when the ferret is young.[1] Lower-protein diets (<35%) have been recommended for older ferrets to prevent chronic interstitial nephritis, although there has been no real evidence to suggest that a high-protein diet causes nephritis in ferrets or that feeding a lower-protein diet either alleviates the condition or stops its progress.[1] Nephritis might actually be caused by unrecognized viral or bacterial infections or other dietary components present in all foods.[1] However, the less active older ferret probably does not need more than 35% protein in his diet and may accept a lower-protein variety of his favorite food.[1] There are geriatric ferret diets on the market,[12] but feeding trials looking at their effectiveness have not been done. If switching foods is a struggle, the possible benefits of the change are outweighed by the stress of the conflict. Some ferrets eat less and lose weight as they age, even when their teeth appear normal and no systemic disease is apparent.[1] It may be that they are losing their sense of smell, because they often eagerly devour their regular pellets mixed with warm water, either alone or with a favorite additive, such as baby food or Nutri-Cal.[1] Because more plaque is deposited on their teeth as a result of the soft diet, their teeth need to be checked and cleaned twice a year.[1,5]

Ferrets with terminal cancer also need special attention to ensure that their nutritional needs are met. This may include extra meals and fortifying supplements.[1] The real secret of maintaining a good quality of life is the faithful care of an owner who is willing to hand-feed an old and/or ill ferret at any and all hours of the day or night.[1]

FEEDING FERRET KITS

If the jill rejects the kits or there are problems with her producing enough milk, supplementation or nursing is required. The formula to use is puppy or kitten milk replacer

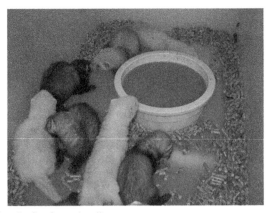

Fig. 5. Kits with bowl of softened pellets.

enriched with cream until the fat content is 20%. The formula that works well is three parts puppy milk replacer (Esbilac, Pet Ag, Hampshire, IL) to one part whipping cream.[24] The kit requires teaching for the first few feedings. Wrap the kit in a towel, with its head protruding. Hold it at an angle that would naturally assume if suckling from the jill. With a drop of milk on it, coax the tip of the cannula (BD Interlink Cannula, Franklin Lakes, NJ) or small animal nipple very gently into the kits's mouth slightly off center.[24] Be prepared to take plenty of time over the first feeding.[24] If the bottle and nipple are not working, use a 1- to 3-mL syringe with a feeding tip or cannula. Dribble the liquid in very gradually and be extremely careful not to choke the infant. Kits drink more if the milk is warm. Start by feeding about 0.5 mL per feed and increase to 1 mL per feed by the end of the first week. A rule of thumb is to let the kit determine the amount. A puppy- or kitten-size bottle and nipple can be used as the kit grows. Soft food can be introduced by 3 to 4 weeks of age. Feed every 2 to 4 hours initially and gradually increase the time interval as the kit matures.[24] At 3 to 4 weeks of age as the eyes open kits can be taught to drink from a low flat dish.[24] In addition to the feeding, the kit needs to be stimulated to urinate and defecate. This can be done by stroking the stomach and back legs. A cotton ball or moistened washcloth can be used to wipe its anogenital area very gentle. Kits start defecating and urinating on their own at about 3 weeks of age. This is about the same time they start to eat mush and move out of the nest box.[24] The mush should be the ferret diet the jill is on, a commercial ferret food moistened with water (**Fig. 5**).

INFLAMMATORY BOWEL DISEASE

It is speculated that inflammatory bowel disease may be associated with current ferret diets, but no definitive studies have been done linking a diet with the development of the disease. Anecdotally, alleviation or moderation of symptoms has been achieved in some ferrets by switching diets, including usage of a novel protein diet (Turkey, Venison, Lamb Meal; Performance Foods). Dietary clay (diosmectite; Smecta; IPSEN Pharmaceuticals, Basking Ridge, NJ) has been shown to have anti-inflammatory effects in colitis in rats at a dosage of 400 mg/kg/day orally.[25] Another dietary edible clay, calcium montmorillonite (Nutramin; California Earth Minderals, Corp, Culver City, CA) has been used in ferrets with some alleviation of symptoms. Studies are needed to clarify the role commercial diets have in this disease and in the treatment of it.

REFERENCES

1. Bell JA. Ferret nutrition. Vet Clin North Am Exot Anim Pract 1999;2(1):169–92.
2. Powers LV, Brown SA. Basic anatomy, physiology, and husbandry. In: Quesenberry KE, Carpenter JW, editors. Ferrets, rabbits, and rodents clinical medicine and surgery. 3rd edition. St Louis (MO): Elsevier Saunders; 2012. p. 1–12.
3. Ball RS. Issues to consider for preparing ferret as research subjects in the laboratory. ILAR J 2006;47(4):348–57.
4. Kupersmith DS. A practical overview of small mammal nutrition. Sem Avian Exotic Pet Med 1998;7(3):141–7.
5. Church RR. The impact of diet on the dentition of the domesticated ferret. Exotic Dvm 2007;9(2):30–9.
6. Eroshin VV, Reiter AM, Rosenthal K, et al. Oral examination results in rescued ferrets: clinical findings. J Vet Dent 2011;48(1):8–15.
7. Lewington JH. Nutrition. In: Lewington JH, editor. Ferret husbandry, medicine and surgery. 2nd edition. Philadelphia: Saunders Elsevier Limited; 2007. p. 57–85.
8. Mazuri reference guide. Brentwood (MO): Mazuri/PMI International Company LLC. Available at: www.mazuri.cl/mazuri-diet-reference-guide.pdf; www.mazuri.com. Accessed February 6, 2013.
9. Matchett C, Marr R, Berard F, et al. The laboratory ferret. A volume in the laboratory animal pocket reference series. Boca Raton (FL): CRC Press; 2012. p. 16–7.
10. Feket SG, Fodor K, Prohaczik A, et al. Comparison of feed preference and digestion of three different commercial diets for cats and ferrets. J Anim Physiol Anim Nutr 2005;89(3–6):199–202.
11. Orcutt CJ. Ferret urogenital diseases. Vet Clin North Am Exot Anim Pract 2003; 6(1):113–38.
12. Hoppes SM. The senile ferret (*Mustela putorius furo*). Vet Clin North Am Exot Anim Pract 2010;13(1):107–22.
13. Carpenter J, Harms C, Harrenstien L. Biology and medicine of the domestic ferret: an overview. J Small Exotic Anim Med 1994;2(4):151–62.
14. Li X, Glser D, Li W, et al. Analyses of sweet receptor gene (Tas1r2) and preference for sweet stimuli in species of carnivore. J Hered 2009;100(Suppl 1): S90–100.
15. Fox JG, McLain DE. Nutrition. In: Fox JG, editor. Biology and diseases of the ferret. 2nd edition. Baltimore (MD): Williams & Wilkins; 1998. p. 149–72.
16. Sundaresan P, Marmillot P, Liu Q, et al. Effects of dietary taurocholate, fat and protein on the storage and metabolism of dietary beta-carotene and alpha-tocopherol in ferrets. Int J Vitam Nutr Res 2005;75(2):133–41.
17. Lederman JD, Overton KM, Hofmann NE, et al. Ferrets (*Mustela putorius furo*) inefficiently convert β-carotene to vitamin A. J Nutr 1998;128(2):271–9.
18. Sanchez J, Fuster A, Oliver P, et al. Effects of β-carotene supplementation on adipose tissue thermogenic capacity in ferrets (*Mustela putorius furo*). Br J Nutr 2009;102:1686–94.
19. Kim Y, Chongviriyaphan N, Liu C, et al. Combined antioxidant (β-carotene, α-tocopherol and ascorbic acid) supplementation increases the levels of lung retinoic acid and inhibits the activation of mitogen-activated protein kinase in the ferret lung cancer model. Carcinogenesis 2006;27(7):1410–9.
20. Kim Y, Chongviriyaphan N, Liu C, et al. Combined α-tocopherol and ascorbic acid protects against smoke-induced lung squamous metaplasia in ferrets. Lung Cancer 2012;75(1):15–23.

21. Liu C, Russell R, Wang XD. Lycopene supplementation prevents smoke-induced changes in p53, p53 phosphorylation, cell proliferation, and apoptosis in the gastric mucosa of ferrets. J Nutr 2006;136:106–12.
22. De Matos RE, Morrisey JK. Common procedures in the pet ferret. Vet Clin North Am Exot Anim Pract 2006;9(2):347–65.
23. Chen S. Advanced diagnostic approaches and current medical management of insulinomas and adrenocortical disease in ferrets (*Mustela putorius furo*). Vet Clin North Am Exot Anim Pract 2010;13(3):439–52.
24. McKimmey V. Ferret kits. In: Gage LJ, editor. Hand-rearing wild and domestic mammals. Ames (IA): Iowa State Press; 2002. p. 203–6.
25. Gonzalex R, Sanchez de Medina F, Martinez-Augustin O, et al. Anti-inflammatory effect of diosmectite in hapten-induced colitis in the rat. Br J Pharmacol 2004; 141:951–60.

Rodent Nutrition
Digestive Comparisons of 4 Common Rodent Species

 CrossMark

Kerrin Grant, MS

KEYWORDS

- Chinchilla • Guinea pig • Hamster • Gerbil • Coprophagy
- Colon separation mechanism (CSM) • Captive diet • Dental issues

KEY POINTS

- Rodents in the suborders Caviomorpha and Myomorpha have dietary differences and different dental formulas.
- Although rodents share a digestive adaptation with lagomorphs, called coprophagy, they use a different mechanism to accomplish it.
- Hamsters differ from other rodents in that they use foregut fermentation, similar to ruminants.
- Hamsters have a digestive adaptation to metabolize oxalates and absorb calcium from them.
- The captive diet of caviomorphs (chinchilla and guinea pigs) is based on grass hay.
- Dental disease is promoted in caviomorphs when the diet lacks adequate fiber and abrasive matter.
- Captive diet of myomorphs (hamsters and gerbils) is based on rodent pellet and seed mix.

INTRODUCTION

The common pocket pets, chinchilla (*Chinchilla lanigera*), guinea pig (*Cavia porcellus*), golden hamster (*Mesocricetus auratus*), and Mongolian gerbil (*Meriones unguiculatus*) represent 2 subgroups of Rodentia: the infraorder Caviomorpha (chinchilla and guinea pig) and suborder Myomorpha (hamster and gerbil). Wild relatives of chinchilla and guinea pig are New World porcupines, nutria, capybara, and degu. Relatives of hamsters and gerbils are rats, mice, voles, and lemmings.

Natural Diet

Caviomorphs
Caviomorphs are rodents that originated in South America (and 1 in North America). Their natural diet is herbivorous and comprises some combination of wild fruit, leaves,

Conflict of Interest: None.
ICU, The Wildlife Center, PO Box 246, Espanola, NM 87532, USA
E-mail address: zoonutrition@msn.com

Vet Clin Exot Anim 17 (2014) 471–483
http://dx.doi.org/10.1016/j.cvex.2014.05.007

and grasses, depending on species. Myomorphs may have herbivorous, granivorous, or omnivorous feeding strategies and consume a diet of seeds, fruit, vegetation, and insects.

Chinchillas are native to the Andes Mountains in South America. There are 2 recognized species: *C lanigera* (long-tailed chinchilla), the progenitor of pet chinchillas, and *Chinchilla chinchilla* (formerly *Chinchilla brevicaudata*), commonly known as the short-tailed chinchilla. Both species are critically endangered in the wild.[1,2] The weight range of wild long-tailed chinchilla is 369 to 493 g for males and 379 to 450 g for females.[3] Domestic male chinchillas weigh up to 600 g and females 800 g.[4]

Consistent with the caviomorph feeding strategy, chinchillas are herbivores, and are considered to be folivorous, opportunistic feeders. Their diet is seasonally varied, consisting of roots, leaves, fruit, berries, bark, alfalfa, grasses, shrubs, and cacti. They prefer dried leaves rather than fresh; succulents and seeds comprise only a small part of the diet.[5] The diet is naturally high in fiber (>66% of the diet), coming from bark, woody stems, and bromeliads. To mimic the wild feeding strategy as closely as possible, the captive diet should contain grass hay as a main dietary component.

Guinea pigs have been domesticated in South America for thousands of years. Little information is available on the specific diet of their wild counterparts; however, they are considered strict herbivores. Habitat studies place them in open grasslands, consisting of short grasses.[6] A captive diet containing grass hay for adults and mixed grass hay/alfalfa for growing pigs and lactating females is appropriate. Adult weight is 700 to 1200 g.[7]

Both the chinchilla and guinea pig have a dental formula of 2 (I 1/1, C 0/0, PM 1/1, M 3/3) = 20. Because they evolved on a diet of fibrous vegetation that constantly wears down teeth, they have open-rooted hypsodont cheek teeth (high crowned with enamel extending past the gum line) that grow continuously throughout their lives.[8-10] Captive animals fed a diet lacking in adequate fiber/abrasive material are prone to malocclusions and other dental issues.[11]

Myomorphs

Hamsters and gerbils are myomorphs and belong to the family Cricetidae. The natural diet of both the Syrian golden hamster and Mongolian gerbil consists of seeds, fruits, grasses, leaves, and insects.[12,13] Adult hamster body weight is 85 to 130 g for males and 95 to 150 g for females. Gerbils weigh 70 to 135 g, with males being slightly heavier than females.[14]

Gerbils naturally inhabit arid and semiarid regions. Because of this, it was once thought they did not require fresh drinking water. Although they consume a predominantly dry diet, they also eat succulents with high moisture content. In captive studies, gerbils maintained on only a dry diet had higher mortalities than animals that were provided with fresh water.[15] It was determined that gerbils consume water from fresh sources and succulent plant matter at an amount comparable with 8% to 13% of their body weight per day (4–10 mL/100 g body weight).[16]

Hamster and gerbil dental formula is 2 (I 1/1, C 0/0, PM 0/0, M 3/3) = 16. Unlike the chinchilla and guinea pig, hamsters and gerbils have brachyodont (low-crowned) dentition with anatomic roots that stop growing after they are fully erupted.[11] This type of dentition is appropriate for a diet consisting mostly of seeds, grains, leaves, and other matter that does not continuously wear on the teeth. In captivity, hamsters and gerbils are less prone to develop dental disease of their molars than their caviomorph relatives.

DIGESTIVE ANATOMY
Chinchilla

Chinchillas are hindgut fermenters and have a large, coiled cecum and sacculated colon.[17] The cecum may contain 23% of the gastrointestinal (GI) matter, which is one-third to one-half that of guinea pigs.[18] The small and large intestine of the chinchilla is 3.5 m long (11.5 feet),[19] which is almost twice as long as in the guinea pig. Total transit time through the GI tract is 12 to 15 hours.[20] Cellulose digestion occurs in the large intestine with production of volatile fatty acids (VFAs), used as an energy source. VFA composition is approximately three-quarters acetic acid, with the remaining 25% split almost equally between butyric and propionic acids.[21]

Guinea Pig

Guinea pigs are also hindgut fermenters with a GI anatomy consisting of a monogastric glandular stomach, large cecum, and colon. The lesser curvature of the stomach is small and forms an angle with the esophagus called an angular notch.[22] Most food leaves the stomach within 2 hours and GI transit time is ~20 hours, with most digestion occurring within the cecum and colon.[23]

The cecum is a large, thin-walled sac between the small and large intestine, filling most of the left ventral abdomen.[22] The cecum may hold 44% to 65% of GI content and total area is 29% larger than the colon.[17,23,24]

Approximately one-third of the total colon length is the proximal colon, in which mucosal folds form a furrow to separate protein and small particles from poor-quality matter. Nutritious material in the proximal colon is transported back to the cecum for further fermentation by bacteria and protozoa, whereas non-nutritious matter is excreted.[22]

Gut flora is mainly gram-positive bacteria, but anaerobic *Lactobacillus* spp, coliforms, yeasts, and *Clostridium* spp may be present in small numbers.[25] The guinea pig is one of the few herbivores that naturally carry *Lactobacillus* in the GI tract. Dietary fiber is needed to maintain normal gut flora populations. Without fiber, gut motility slows down, and the pH of the cecum changes; fermentation rate is then affected, and indigestion results. The fiber requirement for guinea pigs in captivity is greater than or equal to 15% of the diet (on a dry matter basis), although a diet closer to 30% to 35% acid detergent fiber (ADF) and crude fiber may be beneficial for gut health. ADF and crude fiber content of common grass hays (eg, timothy, orchard, and oat hay) is ~30% to 39%.

Hamster

Unlike other rodents, hamsters have a distinctly compartmentalized stomach consisting of a forestomach (pregastric section) and glandular stomach (gastric pouch). The two compartments of the stomach are separated by a sphincterlike muscle constriction.[26] The forestomach is analogous to the rumen, although it comprises only 37% of the total stomach.[26,27] It is lined with keratinized epithelium, like that found in ruminants and pseudoruminants.[26] Gut flora in the hamster forestomach is also comparable with those found in cattle and sheep.[28] Fermentation takes place in the forestomach and produces VFAs that may be absorbed and used as an energy source.[26] Acetic acid is the main VFA produced (75%–80% of total), with the remaining split almost equally between butyric and propionic acids.[26] The hamster's GI tract is considered the simplest example of a polygastric digestive system.[29]

The benefit of the separate forestomach is that it acts as a buffer to varying protein quality, thereby allowing the hamster to be less dependent on protein quality than a species like the rat.[30] When urea was added to a controlled hamster diet, retention was 71%, whereas rats fed the same diet did not retain, or use, urea as a protein source.[28] Although hamsters are less dependent on protein quality than other rodents, because the forestomach is only one-third of the total stomach area, they are more protein-quality dependent than ruminants.

Gerbil

There are many species of wild gerbils. The diet is generally omnivorous, although some species are more granivorous (seed dependent), whereas others consume mainly green vegetation.[13] Like other rodents, gerbils have a large cecum and colon, although granivores tend to have lower gut capacity and smaller cecum and colon that true herbivores.[31] The cecum is 3% to 5% of the body weight. The small intestine of granivores, such as the Mongolian gerbil, is longer than in more herbivorous species, with the small intestine being 48% and large intestine 40% of the total intestinal length. Gerbils have the ability to lengthen the GI tract in response to increased dietary fiber.[31]

COPROPHAGY

Hindgut fermenters, such as rodents, have large energy demands based on body mass that are greater than for larger species (eg, horse). A small rodent requires considerably more food to meet its energy demands, and passage rate through the GI tract is much faster, than a horse on the same diet, but the fermentation rate is similar for the two species.[24] Therefore, fermentation is too slow and food retention times too short for the rodent to receive a sufficient amount of energy to sustain itself. An adaptation to deal with this dilemma is microbial fermentation in the cecum and proximal colon. Fermentation combines with autoenzymatic digestion in the foregut to allow small herbivores to recycle nutrients for additional absorption.[24] This adaptation is commonly called coprophagy and benefits small herbivores by allowing them to consume fiber without energy intake restrictions.[32]

Coprophagy is possible in herbivorous hindgut fermenters because of a colonic separation mechanism (CSM) in the digestive tract that separates bacteria and small particles from more indigestible matter. The CSM allows rapid transport of less digestible food while retaining microorganisms and easily digested food particles in the enlarged cecum for fermentation and microbial reproduction.[33,34]

There are 2 general types of CSM:

1. Wash-back: found in lagomorphs. It has short particles, long fluid retention time, and produces 2 distinct types of feces: the typical hard pellet that is excreted, and the soft cecotrophs that contain high levels of nitrogen and certain vitamins that are consumed for additional absorption of those nutrients. This type of CSM has a structure in the proximal colon that allows fluid, bacteria, and small particles to be washed back into the cecum.[34]
2. Mucus trap: found in rodents and some species from other orders. There is a colonic furrow that allows mucus and bacteria to be trapped and transported back to the cecum via antiperistalsis movement at the bottom of the furrow. Less nutritious food matter continues to the distal colon for excretion.[18,24,35,36] Unlike the wash-back system, the mucus trap has simultaneous excretion of fluid and particle passage. Because of this, there may be little visual difference between the excreted feces and the nutrient-dense pellets that are reingested.

There are minor differences between the mucus trap CSM of caviomorphs (guinea pigs and chinchilla) and myomorphs (hamsters and gerbils), although they work in a similar fashion. The differences may be associated with food composition, because myomorphs typically consume a more granivorous or omnivorous diet than the herbivorous caviomorphs. One main difference between the two groups is that in caviomorphs, the nitrogen content (milligrams per gram of dry matter) of cecotrophs is considerably higher than that found in cecal contents (26%–52%) whereas in myomorphs, there is very little difference (5%–6%).[18,37]

The mucus-trap CSM has slower bacterial extraction from the colonic digesta plug than the wash-back system and therefore requires a longer colon to achieve a sufficient degree of bacterial extraction.[24] In rodents, the slower, less complete removal of bacteria in a larger colon allows increased digestibility of fiber. When coprophagy was restricted in guinea pigs, animals showed decreased apparent digestibility of dry matter, organic matter, crude protein, fat, and fiber, as well as increased mineral excretion (100%–200%).[38]

Lagomorphs are more selective feeders than rodents, so require less fiber digestion. The wash-back system and smaller colon therefore create a lighter digestive system, which may be advantageous to species reliant on speed as a method to escape predation.[24] Many rodents use other methods to escape predation (eg, hiding) so the extra weight associated with a larger digestive tract may not be a hindrance. The ability to digest fiber more thoroughly is advantageous in that it allows species to consume poorer quality forage, and therefore opens habitats for exploitation.

A study on different dietary fiber levels in Mongolian gerbils indicated that they did not have CSM but were able to adjust the capacity of the digestive tract to accommodate greater qualities of low-quality food.[31]

OXALATE METABOLISM

Soluble calcium oxalates occur in a variety of plants and are toxic to animals because the oxalates bind with, and prevent absorption of, calcium. Mammalian enzymes do not typically catabolize oxalates but they may be degraded by microbial action in ruminants.[39] Soluble oxalates are also metabolized in some rodents, including hamsters, pack rats, and sand rats.[40]

Pack rats, a species related to hamsters (both belong to the family Cricetidae), consume a diet containing high levels of oxalates (eg, prickly pear and mesquite) and have developed the ability to dissociate calcium ions from the oxalates, which allows calcium absorption and use.[40]

In a study investigating calcium metabolism in hamsters fed oxalates, most of the oxalates were degraded in the intestine, presumably through microbial action, and excreted in the urine.[41] Hamsters were able to absorb calcium by dissociating calcium ions from oxalates, similar to that seen in pack rats, which may reflect an adaptation to a natural diet low in calcium/high in oxalates.[41] Note that white rats, which belong to the family Muridae, were not able to absorb calcium from oxalates when fed the same diet as hamsters, indicating that they did not have a similar adaptation.[41]

CAPTIVE DIET

Table 1 shows the general nutritional requirements for the four rodent species mentioned in this article. For the nutrients listed, the requirements for all 4 species are similar, with the exception of gerbils, which require less dietary fiber. In addition, guinea pigs require dietary vitamin C, and chinchillas may benefit from supplementation for dental health (discussed later).

Table 1
Nutrient requirement for chinchilla, guinea pig, hamster, and gerbil

	Chinchilla[40,42]	Guinea Pig[23,25]	Hamster[28,30,41–44]	Gerbil[29,31,43–46]
Crude protein (%)	16–20	10–16 (adult) 18–20 (growth)	16–20	16 (adult) 17–25 (growth)
Fat (%)	2–5	NA	4–5	2–5
Fiber (%)	15–35	≥15	≥15	6–10
Calcium (%)	0.60	0.80	0.60	0.50
Phosphorus (%)	0.40	0.40	0.35	0.30
Vitamin A (IU/kg)	NA	6.6	1.1	0.7
Vitamin C (mg/kg)	NA	200	NA	NA

Abbreviation: NA, not available.

Chinchilla

- Crude protein deficiency can cause poor hair coat and unthrifty, dry skin[42]
- High-moisture fruits/vegetables can cause bloat
- Sweets and dried fruit (eg, raisins) can cause diarrhea and diabetes
- Coarse hay (alfalfa, orchard grass, timothy, blue grasses) with 14% to 16% crude protein prevents tooth overgrowth[42]
- Long-stemmed hay maintains proper GI function
- Alfalfa should be given to growing and pregnant/lactating animals only
- Chinchilla pellets: offer 1 to 2 tablespoons (20 g/d)
- Mixed greens: offer 1 to 2 teaspoons (5–10 g/d)
- Avoid diets high in pellets, rolled oats, shredded wheat, peanuts, and raisins
- Safe treats[42]:
  ○ Mountain ash berries, fruit tree twigs, dried rose hips, marshmallow root, and dried herbs
- Safe wood[42]:
  ○ Fruit trees that bear seeds (apple, pear, grape); elderberry, bamboo, cottonwood, crab apple, dogwood rose, elm, hazelnut, kiwi, mulberry, willow, and manzanita
  ○ Do not give branches from conifers and citrus wood: they contain resin oils and phenols, which are toxic to rodents
- Require fresh water daily

Guinea Pig

- Offer high-quality guinea pig pellets (one-eighth of a cup per day): must contain vitamin C (200 mg/kg diet or 10–20 mg/pig/d)
- Offer timothy hay ad lib for guinea pigs more than 1 year of age, and alfalfa for young and pregnant/lactating animals
- Offer up to 1 cup of chopped vegetables (eg, broccoli, yam, carrots) and mixed greens (eg, kale, parsley, beet greens) per day
- A small amount of kiwi and/or orange may be given every day for vitamin C
- Require fresh water daily

Hamster

- Offer 10 to 14 g/d of commercial hamster diet (mixture of pelleted diet and seed mix)

- Can offer small amount of fresh vegetables, fruit, and greens 3 times a week
  - Fruit: apple, berries, pear, and plum
  - Vegetables: broccoli, cauliflower, carrots, green beans, asparagus, and zucchini
  - Greens: kale, turnip greens, mustard greens, beet greens, dandelion greens, parsley
- Offer small sticks or branches from fruit-bearing trees and other hard commercial snacks for chewing (for dental health)
- Require fresh water daily

Gerbil

- Offer a diet consisting of 5 to 6 g (8–10 g diet/100 g body weight) hamster/gerbil mix and rodent block per day.
- No need to provide hay in the diet.
- Offer greens and vegetables (carrots, broccoli, mixed salad greens, and pesticide-free dandelion greens) as occasional treats.
- Avoid raw kidney beans, raw potato, onion, potato leaves, or rhubarb leaves.
- Sunflower seeds and peanuts should be avoided because they make animals prone to obesity. In addition, both items are deficient in essential amino acids.
- Require fresh water daily (or vegetables/greens with high moisture content).

NUTRITIONALLY RELATED HEALTH ISSUES
Chinchilla

1. Esophageal choke: occurs from eating raisins, fruit, and nuts.[17]
2. Bloat/gastric tympany: overeating fresh clover, sudden change in diet, especially change to high levels of carbohydrates.[17]
3. Gastric trichobezoars: result of fur chewing and lack of dietary fiber. Increase hay in diet.[17]
4. Constipation: lack of dietary fiber. Can give carrots, apples, greens; discontinue raisins, seeds, and nuts.
5. Diarrhea: caused by diet containing too much fresh vegetable matter; lack of dietary fiber/gut stasis leads to bacterial overgrowth in the GI tract.
6. Constipation: lack of dietary fiber, lack of exercise, obesity.
7. Intestinal torsion, intussusception, and impaction of cecum and/or colon: signs are depression, painful/distended abdomen; needs immediate veterinary intervention.[17]
8. Anorexia may be caused by[47]:
   a. Improper diet
   b. Molar malocclusion
   c. Excessive heat
   d. Respiratory infection/pneumonia
   e. Foreign body obstruction
   f. Lack of exercise/GI stasis
   g. Systemic infection
   h. Trauma/stress
9. Dental issues:
   - The incisors of adult chinchilla are naturally yellow/orange in color. Young are born with white teeth, but white teeth in adults are an indication of calcium or vitamin D deficiency

- Tooth overgrowth may be result of dietary calcium and phosphorus imbalance:
  - Hypercalcemia/hypophosphatemia may be seen in serum Ca and P.[9]
  - Increased serum calcium may result from hyperparathyroidism, or excess dietary vitamin D or calcium.[48,49]
  - Increased calcium can lead to[50–52]: anorexia → lower food intake → reduces mastication → reduced tooth wear.
  - Hypophosphatemia may be caused by[53]:
    - Dietary phosphorus deficiency
    - Dietary vitamin D deficiency
    - Hyperparathyroidism
  - Hypophosphatemia can lead to:
    - Anorexia
    - Tooth decay
    - Ossification disorders
      - Osteomalacia
      - Bone demineralization
      - Osteoporosis
  - Increased serum calcium and magnesium, along with low phosphorus, have been associated with dental overgrowth in chinchilla.[9] **Table 2** shows the normal range of calcium phosphorus and magnesium serum values.
- Tooth overgrowth commonly occurs from inadequate tooth wear (lack of coarse fiber in the diet)[58]
  - Signs of tooth overgrowth[9]:
    - Initial stage: drooling and anorexia, followed by watery eyes. Incisors may be misplaced and elongated, with sharp edges on cheek teeth.[50,59]
    - More advanced stage: elongated tooth roots that are visible on radiographs (roots reach beyond bone surface); osteitis and abscesses.[58,60]
  - The natural chinchilla diet is composed of dry plant components, which promote tooth wear, as does minerals in soil consumed with vegetation.
  - Pelleted diet in captivity is not hard enough to promote appropriate tooth wear, and therefore leads to dental issues.
  - Hay must be included in the diet daily (eg, timothy, orchard grass, oat hay). Hay cuttings after the first of the season are coarser (depending on number of cuttings typical in a given region), because fiber content increases. Midseason-cut hay may be beneficial to chinchilla in that it better matches the fiber content of the natural diet, as well as providing abrasive material to promote dental health.
  - Vitamin C helps prevent dental disease by keeping connective tissue around tooth sockets firm.[20]
    - Rose hips and kiwi are good sources of vitamin C
    - Provide diet with 150 to 200 mg vitamin C per day

Table 2
Comparison of serum calcium phosphorus and magnesium values

	Chinchilla[9,54–56]	Guinea Pig[56,57]	Hamster[56]	Gerbil[56]
Calcium (mg/dL)	5.4–12.02	8.2–12.0	10.4–12.3	3.7–6.0
Phosphorus (mg/dL)	4.0–8.0	3.0–7.6	5.3–6.6	3.7–7.1
Magnesium (mg/dL)	3.3–5.0	1.75–3.89	2.2–2.5	NA
Ca:P ratio	1.4–1.5:1	1.6–2.7:1	~2:1	0.8–1:1

Guinea Pig

1. Anorexia[20]:
   a. Malocclusion
   b. Hindgut dysbiosis (change in microflora and motility)
   c. Dental disease
2. Diarrhea[20]:
   a. Primary to GI disease
   b. After other disease
      i. Diet
      ii. Stress
      iii. Illness
      iv. Anesthesia
      v. Reproduction
      vi. Antibiotics: disrupt gut flora
3. Vitamin C deficiency[20]:
   a. Require 200 mg/kg diet or 10 to 20 mg/pig/d
   b. Signs:
      i. Hind leg weakness
      ii. Gum inflammation
      iii. Rough hair coat
      iv. Bleeding in joints/under the skin
4. GI ileus[20]
   a. Malfunction of the digestive tract caused by decreased gut motility
   b. Caused by lack of dietary fiber: increasing dietary fiber improves gut motility
   c. Signs:
      i. Decreased appetite
      ii. Bloated/distended abdomen
      iii. Lethargy
      iv. Decreased volume/size of feces
5. Enteritis: intestinal inflammation associated with toxins[20]
   a. Caused by low-fiber/high-starch diet
      i. Promotes gut hypomotility
      ii. Changes intestinal pH
      iii. Changes gut flora
      iv. Allows overgrowth of pathogenic bacteria
   b. Signs:
      i. Soft stool
      ii. Hunched dorsum
      iii. Inactivity
      iv. Gas
      v. Abdominal pain
6. Urolithiasis: urinary crystals/stones[20]
   a. Can form from an imbalance of calcium and phosphorus
   b. Caused by:
      i. Natural diet high in calcium
      ii. Vitamin D or magnesium deficiency
      iii. Feeding greens high in oxalates (binds with calcium and decreases absorption)
      iv. Feeding grains high in phosphorus
         • Inverse Ca/P ratio causes urinary stones and tissue calcification

Hamsters

1. Colocolic intussusception (IN)[61]:
   - Proximal portion of intestine telescopes into an adjacent distal portion of intestine.
   - Decreased mucus production in colon.
   - Occurs in hamsters fed high levels of sucrose (65% of diet), which alter gut motility:
     o Normal hamster experimental diets contain 10% sucrose
     o Condition resolved when starch was substituted for sucrose
     o Sources of fat in diet have no impact on IN
   - Excess dietary sucrose may cause water to be retained in the colon by osmosis, causing diarrhea and precipitating IN.
   - Mucus production in colon is reduced in IN, which may cause fecal bolus with poor motility to be a source of IN.
   - Reduced bile secretion and distended gall bladder reduces fat digestion, which decreases intestinal transit time and increases fecal fat content.
   - Signs:
     a. Lethargy
     b. Anorexia and weight loss
     c. Diarrhea
     d. Gall bladder distention
     e. Steatorrhea (20% higher fecal fat output)
     f. Ileal-cecal hemorrhage and ileal-cecal spasms
     g. Liver and pancreas weight lower than in healthy hamsters, but gall bladder grossly distended with bile
2. Dental issues:
   - Not as prone to cheek teeth malocclusions as caviomorphs.
   - Periodontal disease may result from diet high in refined sugar or soft foods.[62] Correct by offering complex carbohydrates and dry food (pelleted diet).
   - Elongated incisors may result from lack of hard items for chewing. Offer commercial hamster wood treats or safe woods appropriate for chinchilla for dental health.

Gerbils

- Gerbils are less prone to nutritionally related health issues than the other species included in this article.
- GI upset and diarrhea may result from imbalanced diet or excess amount of fruit (sugar) and/or high-moisture foods.
- May develop dental disease and obesity when an imbalanced or homemade diet is provided.
- May develop dental issues similar to hamsters if not allowed to chew on hard surfaces (eg, wood).

REFERENCES

1. D'elia G, Teta P. *Chinchilla lanigera*. In: IUCN 2013. IUCN red list of threatened species Version 2013.2. 2008. Available at: http://www.iucnredlist.org. Accessed December 21, 2013.
2. D'elia G, Ojeda R. *Chinchilla chinchilla*. In: IUCN 2013. IUCN red list of threatened species Version 2013.2. 2008. Available at: www.iucnredlist.org. Accessed December 21, 2013.

3. Jimenez JE. Bases biologicas para la conservacion y manejo de la chinchilla chilena silvestre: proyecto conservacion de la chinchilla chilena (*Chinchilla lanigera*). Final report. Santiago (Chile): Corporacion Nacional Forestal–World Wildlife Fund; 1990.

4. Neira R, Garcia X, Scheu R. Análisis descriptive del comportamiento reproductivo y de crecimiento de chinchillas (Chinchilla laniger Gray) en confinamiento. Avances en Producción Animal (Chile) 1989;14:109–19.

5. Cortes A, Miranda E, Jimenez JE. Seasonal food habits of endangered long-tailed chinchilla: the effect of precipitation. Mamm Biol 2002;67:167–75.

6. Cassini MH, Galante ML. Foraging under predation risk in the wild guinea pig: the effect of vegetation height on habitat utilization. Ann Zool Fennici 1992;29: 285–90.

7. Vanderlip S. The guinea pig handbook. Hauppauge (NY): Barron's Pet Handbooks; 2003. p. 13.

8. Williams SH, Kay RF. A comparative test of adaptive explanations for hypsodonty in ungulates and rodents. J Mammal Evol 2001;8:207–29.

9. Muszczynski Z, Sulik M, Ogonski T, et al. Plasma concentration of calcium, magnesium and phosphorus in chinchilla with and without tooth overgrowth. Folia Biol (Krakow) 2010;58(1–2):107–11.

10. Crossley D. Clinical aspects of rodent dental anatomy. J Vet Dent 1995;12(4):131–5.

11. Legendre LF. Malocclusions in guinea pigs, chinchillas and rabbits. Can Vet J 2002;43(5):385–90.

12. Gattermann R, Fritzsche P, Neumann K, et al. Notes on the current distribution and the ecology of wild golden hamsters (Mesocricetus auratus). J Linn Soc Lond Zool 2001;254:359–65.

13. Naumova EI, Zharova GK, Christova TY. Isolating structures of gerbils' digestive tract (Gerbillidae, Rhombomys, Meriones) and their functional significance. Biol Bull 2011;38(4):379–85.

14. NRC. Nutrient requirements of laboratory animals. 4th edition. Washington, DC: National Academy Press; 1995. p. 125, 140.

15. McManus JJ. Early postnatal growth and the development of temperature regulation in the Mongolian gerbil, Meriones unguiculatus. Comp Biochem Physiol A 1971;43:959–67.

16. McManus JJ. Water relations and food consumption of the Mongolian gerbil, Meriones unguiculatus. J Mammal 1972;52:782–92.

17. Donnelly TM. Disease problems of chinchillas. In: Quesenberry KE, Carpenter JW, editors. Ferrets, rabbits and rodents, clinical medicine and surgery. 2nd edition. St Louis (MO): WB Saunders; 2004. p. 255–65.

18. Holtenius K, Bjornhag G. The colonic separation mechanism in the guinea pig (Cavia porcellus) and the chinchilla (Chinchilla laniger). Comp Biochem Physiol A 1985;82:537–42.

19. Williams CSF. Practical guide to laboratory animals. St Louis (MO): CV Mosby; 1976. p. 3–11.

20. Johnson-Delaney CA. Anatomy and physiology of the rabbit and rodent gastrointestinal system. Proceedings of Association of Avian Veterinarians, Association of Exotic Mammal Veterinarians (AEMV) Sessions. 2006. p. 9–17.

21. Krishnamurti CR, Kitts WD, Smith DC. Digestion of carbohydrates in the chinchilla (Chinchilla lanigera). Can J Zool 1974;10:1227–33.

22. O'Malley B. Clinical anatomy and physiology of exotic species: structure and function of mammals, birds, reptiles and amphibians. London: Elsevier Saunders; 2005.

23. Manning PJ, Wagner JE, Harkness JE. Biology and diseases of guinea pigs. In: Fox JG, Cohen BJ, Lowe FM, editors. Laboratory animal medicine. Orlando (FL): Academic Press; 1984. p. 149–77.

24. Bjornhag G. Adaptations in the large intestine allowing small animals to eat fibrous foods. In: Chivers DJ, Langer P, editors. Digestive systems of mammals. Melbourne (Victoria): Cambridge University Press; 1994. p. 287–309.

25. Harkness JE, Wagner JE. Biology and medicine of rabbits and rodents. 4th edition. Media (PA): Williams and Wilkins; 1995.

26. Hoover WH, Manning CL, Sheerin HE. Observations on digestion in the golden hamster. J Anim Sci 1969;28:349–52.

27. Warner RG, Flatt WP. Anatomical development of the ruminant stomach. In: Dougherty RW, editor. Physiology of digestion in the ruminant. Washington, DC: Butterworth; 1965. p. 24–38.

28. Ehle FR, Wagner RF. Nutritional implications of hamster forestomach. J Nutr 1978;108:1047–53.

29. Matsumoto T. Nutritive value of urea as a substitute for feed protein. I. Utilization of urea by the golden hamster. Tohoku J Agrie Res 1955;6:127–31.

30. Banta CA, Warner RG, Robertson JB. Protein nutrition of the golden hamster. J Nutr 1975;105:38–45.

31. Pei YX, Wang DH, Hume ID. Effects of dietary fibre on digesta passage, nutrient digestibility and gastrointestinal tract morphology in the granivorous Mongolian gerbil (*Meriones unguiculatus*). Physiol Biochem Zool 2001;74(5): 742–9.

32. Van Soest PJ. Allometry and ecology of feeding behavior and digestive capacity in herbivores: a review. Z Biol 1996;15:455–79.

33. Bjornhag G, Snipes RL. Colonic separation mechanism in lagomorph and rodent species – a comparison. Zoosystem Evol 1999;75(2):275–81.

34. Franz R, Kreuzer M, Hummel J, et al. Intake, selection, digesta retention, digestion and gut fill of two coprophageous species, rabbits (*Oryctolagus cuniculus*) and guinea pigs (*Cavia porcellus*) on a hay-only diet. J Anim Physiol Anim Nutr 2011;95:564–70.

35. Takahashi T, Sakaguchi E. Role of the furrow of the proximal colon in the production of soft and hard feces in nutrias (*Myocastor coypus*). J Comp Phys B 2000; 170:531–5.

36. Takahashi T, Sakaguchi E. Transport of bacteria across and along the large intestinal lumen of guinea pigs. J Comp Phys B 2006;176:173–8.

37. Sperber I, Bjornhag G, Ridderstrale Y. Function of proximal colon in lemming and rat. Swedish J Agri Res 1983;13:243–56.

38. Hintz HF. Effect of coprophagy on digestion and mineral excretion in the guinea pig. J Nutr 1969;99:375–8.

39. Dodson ME. Oxalate ingestion studies in the sheep. Aust Vet J 1959;35:225–33.

40. Morris MP, Garcia-Rivera J. The destruction of oxalates by the rumen contents of cows. J Dairy Sci 1955;38:1169.

41. Shirley EK, Schmidt-Nielsen K. Oxalate metabolism in pack rat, sand rat, hamster and white rat. J Nutr 1967;91:496–502.

42. Hoefer HL, Crossley DA. Chinchillas. In: Meredith A, Redrobe S, editors. Manual of exotic pets. Quedgeley (United Kingdom): British Small Animal Medical Association; 2002. p. 65–75.

43. Knapka JJ, Judge FJ. The effects of various levels of dietary fat and apple supplements on growth of golden hamsters (*Mesocricetus auratus*). Lab Anim Sci 1974;24:318–25.

44. Stralfors A. Inhibition of dental caries in hamsters. V. The effect of dibasic and monobasic phosphate. Odontol Revy 1961;12:236–56.
45. Arrington LR, Ammerman CB, Franke DE. Protein requirement of growing gerbils. Lab Anim Sci 1973;23:851–4.
46. Hall SM, Zeman FJ. The riboflavin requirement of the growing Mongolian gerbil. Life Sci 1968;7:99–106.
47. Corriveau LA. Chinchilla wellness. Purdue Univ. College. 2010. Available at: www.vet.purdue.edu/vth/sacp/documents/ChinchillaWellness.pdf. Accessed November 28, 2013.
48. Hernandez-Fernandez M, Pelaez-Compomanes P. Ecomorphological characterization of Murinae and Cricetidae (Rodentia) from the Iberian Plio–Pleistocene. Coloquios de Paleontologia 2003;1:237–51.
49. Baranowski P, Wojtas J, Cis J, et al. Value of craniometrical traits in chinchillas (Chinchilla laniger) skulls considering teeth defects. Bull Vet Inst Pulawy 2008; 52:271–80.
50. Crossley DA, Del Mar Miguelez M. Skull size and cheek – tooth length in wild-caught and captive-bred chinchillas. Arch Oral Biol 2001;46:919–28.
51. Liesgang A, Hatt JM, Wanner M. Influence of different dietary calcium levels on the digestibility of Ca, Mg and P in Hermann's tortoises (Testudo hermanni). J Ani Phy & Ani Nutr 2007;91(11–12):459–64.
52. Sone K, Koyasu K, Tanaka S, et al. Effect of diet on the incidence of dental pathology in free living caviomorph rodents. Arch Oral Biol 2005;50:323–31.
53. Arnold WH, Gaengler P. Quantitative analysis of the calcium and phosphorus content of developing and permanent human teeth. Ann Anat 2007;189:183–90.
54. Silva TO, Kreutz LC, Barcellos LJ, et al. Reference values for chinchilla (Chinchilla laniger) blood cells and serum biochemical parameters. Ciência Rural, Santa Maria 2005;35(3):602–6.
55. Smielewska-Los E. Alimentary system disorders in the chinchilla. Mag Wet 2000; 9:8–9 [in Polish].
56. Hillyer EV, Quesenberry KE. Ferrets, rabbits and rodents, clinical medicine and surgery. Philadelphia: WB Saunders; 1997. p. 257, 297.
57. Rabe H. Reference ranges for biochemical parameters in guinea pigs for the Vettest®8008 blood analyzer. Tierarztl Prax Ausg K Kleintiere Heimtiere 2011; 39(3):170–5.
58. Komsta R. Radiographic dental diagnostics of rodents. International Stomatological Symposium. Lublin, 2008. p. 13–6. [In Polish].
59. Sulik M, Seremak B, Muszczynski Z, et al. Cases of dental disease in farm chinchillas (Chinchilla laniger). Zesz Nauk Przegl Hod 2004;72:141–7 [in Polish].
60. Crossley DA, Jackson A, Yates J, et al. Use of computed tomography to investigate cheek tooth abnormalities in chinchillas (Chinchilla laniger). J Small Anim Pract 1998;39:385–9.
61. Cunnane SC, Bloom SR. Intussusception in the Syrian golden hamster. Br J Nutr 1990;63:231–7.
62. Mitchell DF. Production of periodontal disease in the hamster as related to diet, coprophagy and maintenance factors. J Dent Res 1950;29:732–9.

Prescription Diets for Rabbits

Laila Maftoum Proença, MV, DVM, MS, PhD*,
Jörg Mayer, DVM, MSc, DABVP (ECM), DECZM (small mammal)

KEYWORDS

- Prescription diets • Rabbit nutrition • Rabbit nutritional disorders
- Rabbit dietary management

KEY POINTS

- Nutrition plays a major role in health, disease prevention, and longevity of pet rabbits.
- Most information about husbandry and nutrition for long-living pet rabbits is based on short-living production animals, and such comparison is not always adequate.
- The concept of therapeutic nutrition is well recognized in dogs and cats and is beginning to increase in companion rabbit medicine.
- Nutritional management can be used in conjunction with drug therapy, and this complementary approach can bring more effective results.
- Prescription diets are available for selected diseases and conditions of pet rabbits.

INTRODUCTION

Rabbits represent a popular companion animal in the United States. The size of the companion rabbit population in 2012 was estimated at 3.2 million by the American Pet Products Manufacturers Association, and the number of households owning rabbits was 1.4 million.[1]

The scientific literature about husbandry and nutrition for production and laboratory rabbits is extensive. However, the same amount of studies and information is not available for longer-living companion rabbits. Most information used for pet rabbits is extrapolated from production animals. Only scarce studies of proper husbandry and nutrition have been conducted for pet rabbits, and important information is still lacking. Despite the popularity of rabbits as companion animals, health problems related to poor nutrition and husbandry are still common and a major reason for visits to veterinarians.

As in dogs and cats, nutrition plays a major role in health, disease prevention, and longevity of rabbits. Diseases can affect the digestion, absorption, or use of a nutrient,

Declaration: Dr L.M. Proenca's residency is funded by Supreme Petfoods.
Department of Small Animal Medicine and Surgery, College of Veterinary Medicine, University of Georgia, 501 DW Brooks Drive, Athens, GA 30602, USA
* Corresponding author.
E-mail address: proenca@uga.edu

and so the content of the food, its form, and the route by which it is given can be altered. Modifying the diet can be used to treat diseases, such as diets designed specially to dissolve uroliths in cats, low-protein and sodium-restricted diets used in renal disorders in dogs and, nutritionally balanced, high-fiber, and low-calorie diets using for treating obesity in dogs.

Dietary management is important for successful treatment of many diseases. The concept of therapeutic nutrition is well recognized in dogs and cats and is beginning to increase among other pet species, including rabbits. Nutritional products can be used in conjunction with drug therapy, and this complementary approach usually brings faster and more effective results.

The purpose of this article is to review selected nutritional disorders of pet rabbits and their immediate-term, short-term, and long-term dietary management. The prescription diets are presented, focusing on their indications and applications for selected rabbit nutritional disorders, such as gastrointestinal (GI) stasis, obstruction and bloat, teeth malocclusion, obesity, urolithiasis, and hypercalcinuria. At the time of writing, no long-term prescription diets for rabbits were available in the US market, but they could be found in different countries. In addition, the most common myths and misconceptions involving rabbit nutrition are addressed. An appreciation of the normal GI physiology is essential for the understanding of this article, and the reader is encouraged to review previously published literature.

SELECTED RABBIT NUTRITIONAL DISORDERS
GI Stasis, Obstruction, and Bloat

GI stasis is the most common disorder in pet rabbits. It can happen as a primary disorder or secondary in conjunction with other disorders. The cause of GI stasis varies, but it is often correlated with inappropriate diet, more specifically, low indigestible fiber intake. However, any illness, painful condition, or stress in the household can trigger an episode of GI stasis.[2,3]

The clinical sings of GI stasis include inappetence, anorexia, abdominal discomfort, teeth gridding, reduction in the size or quantity of fecal pellets, and absence of fecal production.[3] The case should be considered as an emergency if the condition exists for 24 hours. GI stasis can rapidly become life threatening when not addressed promptly. Low levels (<12.5%) of indigestible fiber in the diet inhibit normal GI peristalsis. Conversely, high levels of digestible fiber lead to abnormal cecal fermentation and inappropriate production of volatile fatty acids, resulting in change in the cecal pH, causing dysbiosis.[4] As a consequence, potentially pathogenic bacteria, normally present in small numbers in the cecum, such as Clostridium sp and Escherichia coli, can overgrow, causing enterotoxemia with diarrhea, which can be associated with a GI bloat.[4]

Another rare but possible disorder is the obstruction of the GI tract with ingested hair or other fibers. If the GI peristalsis is normal, the ingested hair is excreted normally with the ingesta. If the GI motility is impaired, the hair can accumulate in the stomach, causing obstruction and compaction. Often, a sick rabbit refuses to drink normally, leading to a mild dehydration, which can contribute to a stomach outflow problem. It is important to rule out obstruction before the beginning of the treatment of GI stasis, such as stimulating GI peristalsis.[5]

When GI stasis occurs, the animal rapidly develops hepatic lipidosis (see obesity section for details); fatal conditions of hepatic lipidosis can develop within 48 hours.[2] When working up these cases, it is important to exclude underlining causes of GI stasis, such as infection and renal or dental disease.[5]

The diagnosis of GI stasis is usually made by the association of detailed clinical history with the physical examination and abdominal radiographs or ultrasonography. Blood biochemistry can be helpful in identifying electrolytes imbalance or organ failure. Aspects of the dietary history such as recent change in the food brand, introduction of new items, treats, fiber content, and hay availability are important and should not be overlooked.[2–4]

Rabbits with GI stasis need to be aggressively treated with fluids, pain medication, and increase of fiber intake, until they start passing feces and eating again. Pain should always be addressed, because it can lead to anorexia and consequent hepatic lipidosis. In case of gas distention or tympany, the stomach can be decompressed with the passage of a nasogastric tube. Prokinetics enhancers, such as metoclopramide and cisapride, may be of benefit to promote motility of the stomach and intestines, if obstruction is not present.[2–4] However, these drugs should not be used until a diagnosis of primary GI stasis has been established and a cause has been found. In our experience, using GI motility enhancers might not be beneficial if the primary cause of the stasis (eg, pain) has not been adequately addressed.

If the animal is starting to eat, high-fiber intake can be provided with the use of ad libitum Timothy hay (~30%–35% fiber). Alternatively, or in association with hay, a prescription diet can also be used. Rabbit Digestive Health Formula (32% fiber) (Supreme Pet Foods, Suffolk, United Kingdom) is an option to increase indigestible fiber intake (long fiber), to stimulate GI motility.

The use of this prescription diet can be beneficial if owner compliance on providing hay is not ideal, because it can also be used in the long-term. A recent study showed that owners are more likely to provide a pelleted diet as a main source of the rabbit concentrate. The survey study, with 102 pet rabbit owners, showed that in 55 of the cases, the owners provided pellets only, as part of the concentrate. In 35 cases, the rabbits were fed rabbit mix, in 10 cases a combination of pellets and mix, and in 2 cases, the rabbits received no concentrates at all.[6]

If the animal is anorexic, special powder formulated diets, high in fiber, such as Critical Care, Critical Care Fine Grind (Oxbow Animal Health, Murdock, NE, USA), Emeraid Herbivore (Lafeber's, Cornell, IL, USA), or RecoveryPlus (Supreme Pet Foods, Suffolk, United Kingdom) can be reconstituted with water and syringe fed to the animal. Some of these formulas can also be given through a nasogastric tube, but this is often limited by particle size and fluidity. When the fiber particles are small enough to pass into the nasogastric tube without clogging it, they are probably small enough to enter the cecum, instead of the colon, where the indigestible (long) fiber increases GI motility. In the cecum, the digestible (small) fiber undergoes fermentation, instead of promoting GI motility.[2,5]

Teeth Malocclusion

Rabbits are highly specialized herbivores, with anatomy and physiology adapted to accommodate their unique diet. The dental formula of a rabbit is 2 (I2/1, C0/0, PM3/2, M3/3) = 28. Their teeth are hypsodont and elodont, with growing rates from 2 to 2.4 mm per week. Because the maxillary and mandibular cheek teeth differ in number, each mandibular tooth occludes with 2 maxillary cheek teeth, except for the first and sixth maxillary teeth. The normal occlusal surface is not an even plane and contains transverse ridges.[7,8]

Diets low in crude fiber can lead to dental malocclusion as well as decreased GI motility. Other causes of malocclusion include genetics, trauma, and infection. Some rabbit breeds, such as dwarf and lop breeds, are more prone to developing dental malocclusion, which is usually seen in very young animals.[7]

Dental malocclusion can be simple, with the presence of dental sharp points only, or can be a serious dental disease complex, occurring in association with periodontal and endodontal disease, such as dental abscesses. Common clinical signs of malocclusion include inappetence, anorexia, dysphagia, sialorrhea, tooth grinding, epiphora, buphthalmos, facial swelling, weight loss, and nasal discharge.[8,9]

For a complete dental evaluation and oral examination, general anesthesia is required. It is best performed using an otoscope, which allows magnification and best lighting. Alternatively, an oral speculum can be used, providing limited visualization. Whenever possible, computed tomography (CT) should be included in the evaluation of the dental disease complex. Skull CT is the gold standard examination to identify concurrent lesions, such as osteomyelitis and abscessation. Alternatively, skull radiographs can be used, offering limited evaluation only, because some lesions can be recognized only on CT.

When addressed early, malocclusions are simple to correct, via coronal reduction using high-speed dental equipment and special burrs. Conversely, chronic and severe presentations may require surgery, such as dental extractions and abscess marsupialization.[8]

Prevention is a key component of the dental malocclusion complex. As for the GI stasis treatment, it is important to provide high indigestible fiber in the diet, with the use of ad libitum Timothy hay or extruded pellets with high crude fiber content (≥18%). Alternatively, or in association with hay, a prescription diet can also be used. Digestive Health Formula (32% fiber) is an option to increase indigestible fiber intake (long fiber) and natural teeth trimming.

In cases in which surgery is necessary, special powder formulated diets, high in fiber, such as Critical Care, Critical Care Fine Grind, Emeraid Herbivore, or Recovery Plus can be reconstituted with water and syringe fed to the animal as a postsurgical supportive treatment. These formulas do not promote natural teeth trimming. The animal should be stimulated to eat Digestive Health Formula or hay as soon as possible, to provide adequate dental wear.

Obesity

Obesity is a recognized problem among pet animals. Dogs and cats are considered obese when they are 10% to 15% more than their optimum weight, and scoring systems are well established for these species. Obesity is not always obvious and easily diagnosed in rabbits. Rabbits' dense and sometimes long coat (eg, angora rabbits) and anatomy (eg, dewlap in females) can make it difficult to determine a precise body condition score (BCS), which is often subjective.

A scoring system has not been rigorously validated for pet rabbits. The Pet Food Manufacture Association (http://www.pfma.org.uk/) offers a guideline for owners to identify the BCS of their pet rabbits. Mullan and Main[6] developed a body scoring system, which is shown in **Table 1** and **Fig. 1**.

The same investigators conducted a survey study with 102 pet rabbits showing that 24 (23%) of the animals had a BCS of 4/5 or higher (fat or obese). Forty animals (39%) were classified with a BCS of 3.5/5, which was not defined by the scale in the study (see **Table 1**), and could possibly be considered overweight.[6]

Obese rabbits are prone to grooming difficulties, sludgy urine, cystitis, parasitic skin disease, perianal soiling from uneaten cecotrophs, fly strike, pododermatitis, pregnancy toxemia, cardiovascular disease, arthritis, GI stasis, and consequent death.[4]

Obese animals are also prone to hepatic steatosis, the accumulation of hepatic lipids. The liver has a central role in lipid metabolism by importing serum free fatty

Table 1
Description of BCS of pet rabbits

BCS	Description
0 (emaciated)	Ribs and spine prominently visible along with other bony protuberances. General appearance of very poor condition
1 (very thin)	Ribs likely to be visible and spine easily visible and very prominent on palpation; generally poor appearance; no dewlap present in females
2 (thin)	Spine likely to be visible but ribs may not be visible, both prominent on palpation; dewlap may or may not have some fill in females
3 (good)	Ribs not visible and spine not easily visible but both palpated easily; generally trim appearance with small dewlap in females
4 (fat)	Ribs and spines not visible but palpated moderately easily; generally rounded appearance; moderate dewlap in females
5 (obese)	Ribs and spine not visible and palpated with difficulty; generally rotund appearance often with large skin/fat folds; large dewlap present in females

From Mullan SM, Main DC. Survey of the husbandry, health and welfare of 102 pet rabbits. Vet Rec 2006;159(4):102; with permission.

acid and synthesizing and exporting lipids and lipoproteins. Hepatic lipid accumulation can be caused, among other things, by increased lipogenesis and increased fatty acid influx.[10]

Chronic hepatic steatosis predisposes to hepatic lipidosis. Hepatic lipidosis occurs as a result of excessive fat mobilization from fat storage sites, particularly in cases of prolonged anorexia (ie, >24 hours). The condition is worse in overweight animals, because they already have a high fat accumulation in the liver. Animals on high fatty diets (recommended fat in the food is 2.5%–4%) have an increased risk of developing hepatic lipidosis and during episodes of anorexia have a 2-fold increase in circulating ketones, when compared with animals fed lower-fat diets.[4]

Obesity-induced hypertension has been shown in New Zealand white rabbits. Rabbits fed an ad libitum high-fat diet, constituted of standard rabbit chow, with 10% added fat, for 8 weeks, had a 47% increase in body weight, 14% increase in mean arterial pressure, and 31% increase in heart rate. Obese rabbits also showed changes in renal function, with increased glomerular filtration rate and a net accumulation of sodium.[11]

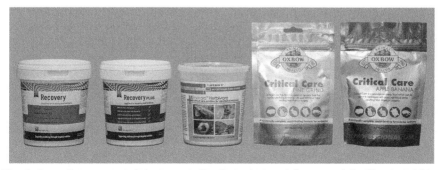

Fig. 1. Immediate-term and short-term diet formulas used for enteral feeding in rabbits. (*Left to right*) Recovery, RecoveryPlus, Critical Care Fine Grind, Critical Care, and Emeraid Herbivore. (*Courtesy of* UGA Veterinary College, Athens, GA.)

Rabbits have been used as a model to better understand arteriosclerosis lesions in humans. Researchers have successfully on caused arteriosclerosis and hepatic lipidosis by adding cholesterol (0.5%) and oil content (peanut oil 2%) to the rabbit diet. It is possible that the same lesions can be caused when pet rabbits are fed high-fat diets.[12]

Treating obese rabbits can be difficult, because it is dependent on the owner's compliance. The use of a prescription diet, such as VetCarePlus Weight Management (Supreme Pet Foods, Suffolk, United Kingdom), can be more effective, because it can be used as the only source of food or in association with Timothy hay. VetCarePlus Weight Management offers a high-fiber (34%) and low-fat (2.5%) diet with reduced calories (1189 kcal/kg). By only changing the diet to a low-calorie food, the owner is able to reduce the calorie intake and promote weigh loss, even when the rabbit is given the same amount of food per day.

Urolithiasis and Hypercalcinuria

Urolithiasis has been reported in rabbits and can occur in any part of the urinary system (bladder, urethra, ureter, and kidney). The cause and pathophysiology of urolithiasis are not completely understood and are likely to be multifactorial. Several factors are suspected to be involved, including nutrition, physiology, anatomy, body condition, lack of exercise, and infection.[13,14]

Calcium metabolism differs in rabbits when compared with other mammals. Calcium absorption in rabbits is not dependable on vitamin D_3, if diet levels are adequate. Passive absorption from the GI tract is the main mechanism for calcium absorption in rabbits. The concentration gradient between the intestinal lumen and blood enables this process, and it is directly affected by the calcium concentration in the diet.[14–16]

Vitamin D_3 is necessary only in cases of hypocalcemia, because it improves calcium absorption. The published requirements for vitamin D_3 are 800 to 1200 IU/kg of body weight. Excess levels of vitamin D_3 (>2300 IU/kg) are associated with disease. Consequently, it is preferable to expose rabbits to sunshine rather than supplement the diet with vitamin D. A short exposure to sunlight seems to be beneficial, because it has been shown that it takes approximately 5 months for serum concentrations of active vitamin D_3 to become undetectable in rabbits on a vitamin D_3-deficient diet.[17,18]

High amounts of calcium in the rabbit's diet lead to hypercalcemia. When supplemented in excess, calcium is excreted by the kidney in the form of calcium carbonate. Fractional urinary excretion of calcium in most mammals is less than 2%, and in rabbits, it is 45% to 60%. The presence of calcium carbonate in the urine gives it the thick, white, and creamy appearance. Because of this unique physiology, the rabbit's normal blood total calcium is usually 30% to 50% higher, when compared with other mammals.[14,15] Readings up to 16 mmol/L (64 mg/dL) can be seen in rabbits fed a high-calcium diet. Care has to be taken not to overinterpret these high calcium levels as a paraneoplastic sign in case other problems exist.

It has been hypothesized that the excess of calcium in the diet, and therefore, excess of calcium carbonate in the urine, can result in urolithiasis.[16] However, this cause has never been proved, and only anecdotal case reports have been published.[19] A recent study showed that rabbits fed a high-calcium diet (2.32%, 1.04%, and 0.83%) for 25 weeks showed no evidence of urolithiasis/calcinosis on radiographs, ultrasonography, or gross pathology. Other factors, such as water intake and level of activity, may be involved in urolithiasis development in rabbit.[13] The effects of calcium in high-cholesterol diets have also been studied. Increased calcium content in diets supplemented with cholesterol has been shown to decrease atherosclerosis lesions in rabbits. Moreover, calcium supplementation of 3% was shown to inhibit atherosclerosis, aorta calcification, and icterus, whereas a calcium-deficient diet of 0.5% promoted these lesions.[12] Clinical signs of urolithiasis include depression, anorexia, weight loss, lethargy, hematuria, anuria, stranguria, hunched posture, grinding of teeth, and urine scald of the perineum. Urolithiasis can also be subclinical or cause constipation as a result of mechanical compression of the intestine by the calculi.[5,14,15,20] Definitive diagnosis of urolithiasis can be achieved with radiographs or ultrasonography. Calculi can sometimes be palpated, as a doughlike mass. Small amounts of amorphous calcium carbonate in the bladder are considered normal in rabbits. Hydroureter or hydronephrosis may occur in combination with urolithiasis and should be evaluated.[21]

Urinalysis is useful in assessing renal function. Normal findings may include crystalluria (calcium oxalate, ammonium phosphate, calcium carbonate, and monohydrate crystals). Proteinuria and hematuria may occur, although trace protein is normally found in the normal rabbit urine. When collected via cystocentesis, urine can be submitted for culture, with E coli and Pseudomonas being known to cause cystitis. Serum or plasma biochemistry and electrolytes (to access renal function), and complete blood count should also be performed.[15]

The treatment of urolithiasis in rabbits is similar to dogs and cats. Before considering surgery, all electrolyte imbalance must be corrected. Hypercalcinuria, when present, should be treated with aggressive fluid therapy. The localization of the calculi determines the best treatment option. If calculi are present in the urethra, catheterization with a 3.5-Fr to 5-Fr soft catheter might help displace the calculi to the bladder using hydropropulsion.[5,15] When the calculi cannot be completely dislodged to the bladder but are dislodged to the cranial urethra, the authors have used a 2.7-mm or 1.9-mm telescope with integrated sheath to visualize and retrieve the calculi with a 1-mm or 1.7-mm atraumatic forceps via cystotomy. If this procedure is not possible, urethrostomy can be performed.

When large calculi are present in the urinary bladder, cystotomy is the treatment of choice. Samples of the bladder wall should be submitted for culture and biopsy. After removal of the calculi, the bladder should be thoroughly flushed via a urethral catheter and abdominal radiographs repeated to ensure complete removal of all calculi. The calculi should be sent for analysis. The most common calculi in the rabbit are composed of calcium carbonate.[20] In association with surgery, treatments with fluids, analgesics, and antibiotic should be provided.

Diet change, to decrease calcium intake, has been suggested to prevent the formation of new calculi.[19] Grass hay and Timothy hay–based pellets, with no alfalfa, have been recommended in cases of urolithiasis. Alternatively, or in association with Timothy hay, a prescription diet can also be used. Rabbit Urinary Tract Health Formula (Supreme Pet Foods, Suffolk, United Kingdom) contains a low calcium content of 0.5%, crude fiber of 28%, and it is based on Timothy hay only (no alfalfa added). The use of a prescription diet facilitates the treatment for the owner and increases the compliance and treatment outcome.

DIETARY MANAGEMENT

Dietary management during periods of anorexia is essential when treating rabbits. Rabbits produce energy during fermentation in the cecum and when cecotrophs are ingested and digested. Cecum fermentation produces volatile fatty acid, which are responsible for 40% of the rabbit calorie requirement. Glucose, lactate, and amylase present in the cecotrophs are also a source of energy for the rabbit.[4,22]

In periods of anorexia, fermentation and volatile acid production do not occur, and therefore, glucose absorption is impaired. The hypoglycemia stimulates lipolysis and mobilization of free fatty acids from the adipose tissue. The free fatty acids from the adipose tissue are transported to the liver, to produce energy from fat metabolism. This process leads to the release of ketone bodies in the blood, causing ketoacidosis and possible death.

Obese animals are more prone to have hepatic lipidosis, because they already have fat accumulation in the liver. Once hepatic lipidosis is established, fatty infiltration occurs in the kidney, and the animal goes into liver and kidney failure.[21]

Nutritional support, along with fluid therapy and acid basic correction, is a key factor in preventing or treating this condition in rabbits. Rabbits with anorexia for more then 24 hours are prone to developing hepatic lipidosis and should receive enteral nutrition, via syringe feedings or nasogastric tubes. Definitive diagnosis of the cause of the anorexia is essential, and a positive energy balance should be provided.[5]

An instant and readily absorbed energy source prevents mobilization of free fatty acids from adipose tissue and development of hepatic lipidosis. Digestible fiber (small fiber) is important for providing nutrients for cecal bacteria. Indigestible fiber is necessary to promote GI motility, although it is difficult to provide when syringe feeding, because of the long fibers. It is important to consider that grinding long fiber to make it small enough to pass through the syringe or tube more likely transforms the particles in to small fiber. Small fiber, or digestible fiber, goes straight to the cecum to be fermented, instead of going to the colon, where it promotes GI motility.[22]

Calculation of Calorie Intake

When parenteral nutrition becomes necessary, the animal's maintenance calorie intake should be calculated and adapted to the animal's condition. Relying on premade charts or recipes can be an inaccurate way of providing true nutrition. The calorie intake should be reevaluated daily, based on the animal's health status and weight.

The maintenance calorie need is calculated based on the animal's weight and metabolism, and than adjusted depending on the animal's physiologic status. It is an individual requirement and should be calculated case by case. To establish the daily maintenance calorie requirement for a rabbit, the animal's basal metabolic rate (BMR) should first be calculated, as follows:

$$BMR = \kappa W^{0.75}$$

BMR = kcal/kg/d; W = weight in kg; κ = kcal/kg constant; for placental mammals the κ constant is 70.

The BMR is the amount of calories necessary only to maintain the rabbit, not taking in to consideration the clinical presentation. The BMR needs to be adjusted for each animal, depending on health status. Usually, the BMR needs to be increased if the rabbit is hypermetabolic and reduced if it is hypometabolic. The BMR is multiplied by an illness factor between 1.2 and 2.0 to account for metabolic needs more than resting. Growth increases the metabolic rate (illness factor of 1.5–3.0). However, starvation and emaciation decrease the metabolic rate, and the animal requires fewer calories than normal (illness factor of 0.5–0.9).[5]

Illness factor × BMR = kcal/d

The daily calorie requirement is matched to the weight of dry enteral powder (in grams), which varies with the product used. The total daily grams of dry powder should be weighed out and divided into small meals spaced throughout the day. Weighing and feeding dry product is more accurate because it is independent of the amount of water being added. More or less water can be added to facilitate passage through a feeding tube and to meet the fluid requirements of the animal.

Enteral feeding and nasogastric tubes

Enteral feeding is a key factor in the prevention and treatment of anorexic rabbits. Dehydration and electrolyte imbalance often accompany anorexia, and the correction of these imbalances should precede enteral feeding. Before force feeding is started, a stomach bloat or outflow problem should be excluded. In many cases of anorexia, the stomach is already distended with ingesta, and adding volume by force feeding is contraindicated.

Syringe feeding is a popular and easy method to provide nutrition to a rabbit. The use of catheter tip syringes facilitates enteral feeding, with the syringe positioned in the diastema. Depending on the animal, the use of smaller syringes, such as 1 or 3 mL, can help provide food. Syringe feeding requires time, because the food needs to be given slowly and in small quantities.

However, critically ill rabbits are often too weak or too nauseous to eat from a syringe. In these cases, the use of nasogastric tubes is recommended. The restriction to this method is the diameter of the tube in relation to the fluidity of the food given. The choice of tube size depends on the size of the rabbit. Usually, 5-F to 8-F (1.7 and 2.7 mm) rubber catheters fit through the nasal cavity of a rabbit. Diet formulations containing long, indigestible fibers, which promote GI motility, typically clot in these size tubes. Blending the formula most likely breaks the fiber and makes it smaller (digestible fiber).[5]

Nasogastric tube can be useful in the critical patient for immediate care, when an instant and readily absorbed energy source is necessary to avoid the development of hepatic lipidosis.

The length necessary to reach the stomach is determined by measuring from the nose to the last rib. A local anesthetic (2% lidocaine gel) can be applied in the rabbit's nose 5 to 10 minutes before insertion of the tube. The head needs to be ventrally flexed but with the neck straight. Sedation may help with tube placement. The tube is passed ventrally and medially into the ventral nasal meatus. Verification of the correct placement of the tube is determined via radiography. Other, more invasive techniques include placement of a percutaneous gastrostomy tube or pharyngostomy tube.[23]

The type of diet used for enteral feeding varies according to the clinical presentation and patient status. The diets can be divided into 3 major categories: immediate-term, short-term, and long-term dietary management. More than 1 type of diet may be used on the same patient, depending on the patient's requirements.

Immediate management diets are the formulas used for the acute care of animals that need a rapid lifesaving elemental nutrition during the critical first days or first week of care (**Fig. 2**). It is ideal to use during periods of anorexia, when hypoglycemia stimulates fat metabolism and consequently, hepatic lipidosis and ketoacidosis. A readily available source of energy (simple sugars), fat, protein, and digestible (short) fiber is necessary to promote cecal fermentation, production of volatile acid production, and consequently, energy (glucose). Because during this phase there is a demand for readily available carbohydrates, the authors recommend stabilizing the rabbit with Emeraid Herbivore, because this is the only product on the US market that contains a small amount of readily available carbohydrates. After the initial period of critical care and stabilization of the patient, the immediate-care diets are no longer recommended, because of the possibility of enterotoxemia, especially in young

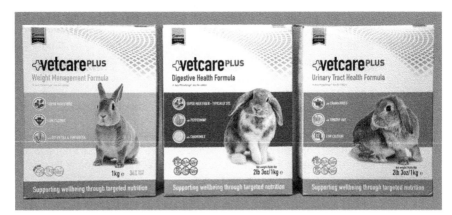

Fig. 2. Prescription diets for long-term nutrition in rabbits. (*Left to right*) Rabbit Weight Management, Rabbit Urinary Tract Health Formula, and Rabbit Digestive Health Formula. (*Courtesy of* UGA Veterinary College, Athens, GA.)

rabbits. Independently, after the acute phase of treatment, it is important to provide a source of indigestible (long) fiber.

Short-term management diets are rich in indigestible (long) fibers, which stimulate GI motility (see **Fig. 2**). These diets are nutritionally complete and can be given as the whole source of diet or in combination with the rabbit's regular diet. Long-term management diets (**Fig. 3**) are specific to determinate health problems, such as obesity, urolithiasis, dental malocclusion, and GI stasis. They are intended to complement medical treatment or prevent the long-term management of a health conditions. It follows the same well-developed concept of long-term prescription diets for dogs

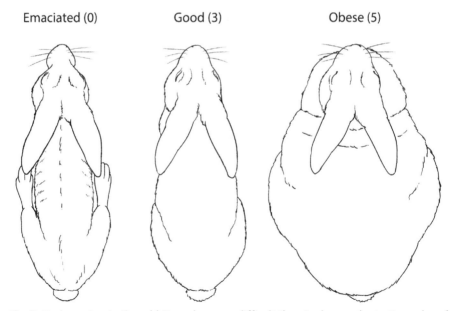

Emaciated (0)   Good (3)   Obese (5)

Fig. 3. Body scoring in the rabbit can be more difficult than in dogs and cats. Examples of the extremes are listed in **Table 1**, with the optimal body score of 3 out of 5 for comparison.

and cats. The list and specifications (provided by the manufacturers) of the immediate-term, short-term, and long-term management diets available in the United States for use with pet rabbits are given in the following sections. **Tables 2–4** show the nutritional requirement for adult rabbits and comparison between analytical constituents and nutritional additives of rabbit prescription diets available in the United States.

Immediate dietary management

Emeraid Herbivore This food is indicated for the immediate care of debilitated animals, which may be fed alone or in combination to provide proper nutrition. It is designed to quickly provide lifesaving elemental nutrition during the critical first week of care (5–7 days). It replenishes the patient's depleted energy, fat, and protein stores. It contains high levels of glutamine and arginine, hydrolyzed proteins, and a high digestible blend of fats and simple carbohydrates for energy. It also contains a balanced amount of omega 3/6 polyunsaturated fatty acids. This diet is indicated for debilitated, cachectic patients, individuals with reduced digestive capacity, patients that require additional calories to maintain or gain weight, and patients needing a minimal number of feedings. It is a highly digestible diet to feed herbivores such as rabbits. This diet contains a high fiber level of 32%, with cellulose as the primary source of fiber. It contains protein levels of 19% and fat levels of 9.5%, with 1.2 kcal/g of dry weight. An additional benefit for this diet is its fine texture, which allows the product to pass through the smaller feeding tubes without clogging them.

Short-term dietary management

i. Recovery diet (Supreme Pet Foods, Suffolk, United Kingdom): for sick and recuperating small herbivores, with a fiber content of 19%, and fructooligosaccharides.

ii. RecoveryPlus diet (Supreme Pet Foods, Suffolk, United Kingdom): intensive nutritional support for the critical care of small herbivores. It is based on Timothy hay,

Table 2
Nutritional requirement for adult rabbits and comparison between analytical constituents of rabbit prescription diets

Diet/Requirement	Protein (%)	Fat (%)	Crude Fiber (%)	Indigestible Fiber (%)	Energy	Crude Ash (%)
Requirement for adult rabbit	12–16	2.5–4	13–20	>12.5	NP	NP
VetCarePlus Weight Management	12	2.5	34	NP	1189 kcal or 4975 kJ/kg	7.5
VetCarePlus Digestive Health Formula	14	3.5	32	NP	NP	7.5
VetCarePlus Urinary Tract Health Formula	14	3.5	28	NP	NP	7.5
RecoveryPlus	18.5	5	25	NP	NP	10
Recovery	17	2	19	NP	NP	7
Emeraid Herbivore	19	9.5	32	NP	1.2 kcal/g dry weight	—
Critical Care	16	3	21–26	NP	24 kcal/tbsp (9 g)	10
Critical Care Fine Grind	16	3	21–26	NP	24 kcal/tbsp	10

Abbreviation: NP, not provided by the manufacturer.

Table 3
Nutritional requirement for adult rabbits and comparison between nutritional additives of rabbit prescription diets

Diet/Requirement	Cl (%)	Cu	I	Vitamin A (IU/kg)	Vitamin Complex B	Vitamin C (mg/kg)	Vitamin D₃ (IU/kg)	O6 (%)	O3 (%)
Requirement for adult rabbit	0.17–0.32	5–20 ppm	0.4–2 ppm	10,000–18,000	0	0	800–1200	NP	NP
VetCarePlus Weight Management	NP	NP	NP	15,000	NP	NP	1500	NP	NP
VetCarePlus Digestive Health Formula	NP	NP	NP	15,000	NP	NP	1500	NP	NP
VetCarePlus Urinary Tract Health Formula	NP	NP	NP	15,000	NP	500	1500	NP	NP
RecoveryPlus	NP	NP	NP	23,000	NP	1200	1400	NP	NP
Recovery	NP	NP	NP	—	NP	—	—	NP	NP
Emeraid Herbivore	NP	NP	NP	—	NP	—	—	4.38	0.37
Critical Care	NP	18 mg/kg	300 mg/kg	19,000	13 µg/kg (B₁₂) plus 60 mg/kg niacin (B₃)	10,000	900	NP	NP
Critical Care Fine Grind	NP	18 mg/kg	300 mg/kg	19,000	13 µg/kg (B₁₂) plus 60 mg/kg niacin (B₃)	10,000	900	NP	NP

Abbreviations: Ca, calcium; Cl, chlorine; Cu, copper; I, iodine; K, potassium; Mg, magnesium; Mn, manganese; Na, sodium; NP, not provided by the manufacture; O3, omega 3; O6, omega 6; P, phosphorus; Se, selenium; unk, unknown; Zn, zinc.

Table 4
Continuation of nutritional requirement for adult rabbits and comparison between nutritional additives of rabbit's prescription diets

Diet/Requirement	Vitamin E	Ca (%)	P (%)	Na (%)	Zn
Requirement for adult rabbit	50 mg/kg	0.5–1	0.4–0.8	0.2–0.25	0.3%–0.6%
VetCarePlus Weight Management	NP	0.8	0.4	0.3	NP
VetCarePlus Digestive Health Formula	NP	0.8	—	0.3	NP
VetCarePlus Urinary Tract Health Formula	NP	0.5	0.4	0.3	NP
RecoveryPlus	80 mg/kg	1	0.6	0.3	NP
Recovery	—	0.8	0.4	0.3	NP
Emeraid Herbivore	—	1	0.39	NP	NP
Critical Care	190 IU/kg	NP	NP	NP	100 mg/kg
Critical Care Fine Grind	190 IU/kg	NP	NP	NP	100 mg/kg

Abbreviations: Ca, calcium; Cl, chlorine; Co, cobalt; Cu, copper; Fe, iron; I, iodine; Mg, magnesium; Na, sodium; NP, not provided by the manufacture; O3, omega 3; O6, omega 6; P, phosphorus; unk, unknown; Zn, zinc.

with long fibers, with a fiber level of 25%. It has a high protein content of 18.5%, with added prebiotics (*Saccharomyces cerevisiae*) and vitamin C (1000 mg/kg). No sugars are added to this product.

iii. Critical Care and Critical Care Fine Grind: this is a complete diet, with 21% to 26% of crude fiber and 16% of crude protein. It is made with Timothy grass. It is indicated for herbivores that are unwilling to eat their normal diet as a result of illness, surgery, or poor nutritional status. Like the other products, this product is a complete diet, which can be reconstituted to be assist fed with a syringe. In our experience, Critical Care can be used for prolonged periods without causing problems to the health of the rabbit.

Long-term dietary management
Prescription diets

Rabbit Weight Management This diet contains reduced energy (1189 kcal/kg of food), with the minimal fat requirement for pet rabbits of 2.5% (compared with 4% fat content of the maintenance diet for the same manufacturer). It is indicated for overweight rabbits to help with weight management. It also contains high crude fiber of 35% (the requirement for pet rabbits is 13%–20%). The fiber is mainly composed of a blend of alfalfa and Timothy hay, with an adequate calcium level of 1% (0.5%–1% is the recommended level) and adequate protein level of 12% (the requirement for an adult pet rabbit is 12%–16%). Composed of extruded pellets, it contains long fiber with no addition of sugars.

Rabbit Digestive Health Formula This extruded diet promotes dental wear with its long fibers and high crude fiber content of 32%. It is indicated for animals with dental malocclusion and GI stasis. Composed of extruded pellets, it contains long fiber with no addition of sugars.

Rabbit Urinary Tract Health Formula This extruded diet contains a low calcium content of 0.5% and still offers a high fiber content of 28%, based on Timothy hay only. It is indicated in cases of urolithiasis in rabbits. Composed of extruded pellets, it contains long fiber with no addition of sugars.

Myths, Misconceptions, and Important Facts

Fiber source and length of particle

Fiber can be classified in 2 major groups: digestible (small or fermentable) or indigestible (long or not fermentable). The main difference is the size, which determines if the fiber particle enters the cecum or the colon.

Indigestible fiber (>0.5 mm) is separated from fermentable components (small particles, <0.3 mm, and fluid) in the proximal colon, and it is rapidly eliminated in hard fecal pellets. Fermentable components are moved back to the cecum, where fermentation occurs, releasing volatile fatty acids that are absorbed as energy source, producing cecotrophs, rich in amino acids and vitamins.[4]

Indigestible fiber (mainly lignin and cellulose) is essential for GI motility. The manufacturing process can influence digestibility; the finer the grinding, the longer the gut transit and cecal retention time and the greater the potential for cecal dysbiosis, as a result of size-dependent separation of particles in the colon. An adequate amount of digestive fiber is important for bacterial fermentation. Indigestible fiber has no effect on the composition of the cecotrophs.[22]

Digestibility of the fiber also affects appetite. Indigestible fiber stimulates appetite and ingestion of cecotrophs. The lower the indigestible fiber content of the diet, the lower the appetite. Lignin, which is almost completely indigestible, when ground to particles smaller than 0.5 mm, passes in to the cecum, instead of going to the cecum to promote intestinal motility.[3,4]

Recommended fiber levels for pet rabbits

Nutritional guidelines for commercial rabbits are well established and studied, including fiber crude content. However, farm rabbits are slaughtered at between 8 and 13 weeks, depending on the weight and breed. They are usually considered satisfactory when they weigh 5 kg.[24] Thus, the diet of a short-living rabbit, which achieves 5 kg in 2 to 3 months, should not be provided to a rabbit that is supposed to live for 8 to 12 years.

Indigestible fiber is important for pet rabbits and it is often overlooked when dealing with commercial animals. Indigestible fiber is important to stimulate GI motility, prevent behavioral problems (eg, fur chewing), provide dental wearing, and stimulate appetite and ingestion of cecotrophs. Fiber levels of 10% to 15% are recommended for commercially produced rabbits but are considered too low as a maintenance diet for pet rabbits. Lowe[25] recommended 13% to 20% of crude fiber, with 12.5% of indigestible fiber for pet rabbits. Fiber levels of 18% or higher are also suggested for companion rabbits.

Crude fiber

Crude fiber refers to the percentage of the original food that remains after boiling in acid and alkali alternately. Crude fiber is mainly a measurement of the lignin and cellulose component of the diet (indigestible fiber). It is not particularly helpful to determine the fermentable or digestible fiber.[4,22]

Carbohydrates and simple sugar

Carbohydrates are an important energy source in the diet. Carbohydrates can be categorized into sugars (monosaccharide), starches (polysaccharide), and digestible fiber (complex carbohydrates present in the plant cell wall).[26]

The general consensus of opinion is that feeding carbohydrates to rabbits has a high risk of causing enterotoxemia. This theory is based on the potential of simple sugars and starches to have a rapid gut transit time (because of incomplete digestion and absorption in the small intestine), enter the cecum (serving as a substrate for bacterial fermentation), and cause pH changes, dysbiosis, and subsequently, enterotoxemia.[4,26]

This process has been described only in young commercial rabbits fed high-carbohydrate, low-fiber diets, and not in adult commercial or pet rabbits. The sensitivity to high-starch diets is controversial in adult rabbits, and the role of starch as a predisposing factor for dysbiosis remains unclear. Adult rabbits seem to digest starch more efficiently than young ones.[27]

The starch provided in the diet has no effect on the chemical composition of cecal contents or on the production or composition of soft and hard feces. There is a difference between the composition of starches, or polysaccharides, and their on the rabbit. Polysaccharides, such as gluco-oligosaccharides (starches that release glucose after hydrolysis), were shown to cause diarrhea in young rabbits. Other starches, such as fructo-oligosaccharides (composed of short chains of fructose, found in many fruits and vegetables) or galacto-oligosaccharides (short chains of galactose, found in the group of prebiotics) do not have the same effect.[2,26]

Diet supplemented with fructo-oligosaccharides was shown to decrease morbidity in rabbits after the introduction of pathogenic E coli. Thus, fructo-oligosaccharides are now included in many rabbit foods.[28]

Molasses

Molasses is used in many commercial diets to improve palatability. Although believed to be high in sugar, molasses is obtained after sugar extraction from sugar cane. It is rich in calcium, iron, and magnesium. One study[29] showed that 15% of molasses in the food was well tolerated by growing rabbits.

Cane molasses contains no protein or dietary fiber and close to no fat. Each tablespoon (20 g) contains 58 kcal, 14.95 g of carbohydrates, and 11.1 g of sugar divided among sucrose (5.88 g), glucose (2.38 g), and fructose (2.56 g). It is rich in calcium, iron, and magnesium.[30]

Vitamin C, vitamin B complex, and vitamin K requirements

Vitamin C is synthesized endogenously in rabbits by the liver, using glucose as a substrate. Therefore, addition of vitamin C is not necessary in the regular rabbit diet, but its use could be indicated during periods of stress or disease (10–50 ppm).[7]

Vitamin B is produced in the rabbit's cecum and is therefore not necessary in the diet, except if the animal is not ingesting the cecotrophs. The production of vitamin B_{12} requires cobalt, which could be a limiting factor in the diet. Vitamin K requirements are unknown for rabbits but should also be produced in the cecum and ingested via cecotrophy.[4,7]

Alfalfa

Alfalfa (Medicago sativa) is a forage legume rich in protein, vitamin A, and calcium. Alfalfa, as well as other legume-rich diets, is believed to predispose to obesity (because of its high protein content) and urolithiasis (because of its high calcium content) in mature nonbreeding animals.

Alfalfa hay crude protein and calcium content are 15% to 20% and 0.9% to 1.5%, compared with 7% to 11% and 0.3% to 0.5% for Timothy hay, respectively.[31] However, alfalfa is high in oxalate, which binds with calcium in the intestine, reducing its absorption (20%–30% of the calcium is in the form of calcium oxalate). The calcium/phosphorus ratio in alfalfa is 5:1. Rabbits are tolerant of a high calcium/phosphorus ratio, and growth rate and bone density are not affected by increasing calcium concentrations to a ratio of 12:1.[4]

Alfalfa can be part of a rabbit's diet. When balanced, the diet can contain small amounts of alfalfa, without predisposing the animal to obesity or urolithiasis. Nevertheless, the high protein content of alfalfa hay can be useful in providing added nutritional demands of lactation, pregnancy, growth, and recovery from certain illness.

Extruded pelleted diet

The process by which pelleted foods are made differs from extruded foods. When pellets are made, the ingredients need to be ground and pressed together, to form a cylinder. Extruded or expanded diets are coarse ground, maintaining longer fiber intact, then cooked to form a paste, which is forced into a shaped diet.

There are 2 types of extrusion processes: cold and hot. In cold extrusion, the temperature of the food remains less than 100°C, whereas during hot extrusion, the ingredients are cooked at a high temperature (>100°C) for a short time. Hot extrusion is used commonly for cereal products, including sugars. Cold extrusion is commonly used for animal feed; because of the low temperature, nutritional losses are generally minimal using this method.

The process of grinding the ingredients can influence particle size, therefore potentially affecting digestibility and rate of passage through the GI tract. Because pellets are ground in small particles, it is possible to incorporate long fiber afterwards, but usually, this process decreases the quality of the fiber and makes the pellet friable (pellets binders can be used to overcome this problem).

The process of extruding food results in a lightweight biscuit. The advantage is that long fiber particles can be incorporated without the pellets becoming friable and disintegrating. The heat treatment applied while cooking the raw ingredients increases starch digestibility. In addition, extruded diets are more palatable and digestible than pelleted rations.

SUMMARY

Dietary management is important for the successful treatment of many diseases and can be used in conjunction with drug therapy. The concept of therapeutic nutrition is well recognized in dogs and cats and is beginning to increase among other pet species, including rabbits. The nutritional component of some rabbit diseases (eg, urolithiasis) is not completely understood, and the clinician should evaluate the use of prescription diets based on the scientific literature and individual needs. Long-term feeding trials are needed to further evaluate the efficacy of prescription diets in rabbits. Prescription diets are now available for selected diseases in rabbits, including diets for immediate-term, short-term, and long-term management.

REFERENCES

1. American Pet Products Manufacturers Association. National pet owners survey. Greenwich (CT): American Pet Products Manufacturers Association; 2012.
2. Harcourt-Brown F. Digestive disorders. Textbook of rabbit medicine. Oxford (United Kingdom): Butterworth Heinemann; 2002. p. 249–91.
3. Oglesbee BL, Jenkins JR. Gastrointestinal diseases. In: Quesenberry KE, Carpenter JW, editors. Ferrets, rabbits and rodents: clinical medicine and surgery. 3rd edition. St Louis (MO): WB Saunders; 2011. p. 193–204.
4. Harcourt-Brown F. Diet and husbandry. Textbook of rabbit medicine. Oxford (United Kingdom): Butterworth Heinemann; 2002. p. 19–51.
5. Paul-Murphy J. Critical care of the rabbit. Vet Clin North Am Exot Anim Pract 2007;10:437–61.

6. Mullan SM, Main DC. Survey of the husbandry, health and welfare of 102 pet rabbits. Vet Rec 2006;159:103–9.
7. Vella D, Donnelly TM. Basic anatomy, physiology, and husbandry. In: Quesenberry KE, Carpenter JW, editors. Ferrets, rabbits and rodents: clinical medicine and surgery. 3rd edition. St Louis (MO): WB Saunders; 2011. p. 157–73.
8. Harcourt-Brown F. Dental diseases. Textbook of rabbit medicine. Oxford (United Kingdom): Butterworth Heinemann; 2002. p. 165–205.
9. Capello V, Lennox AM. Small mammal dentistry. In: Quesenberry KE, Carpenter JW, editors. Ferrets, rabbits and rodents: clinical medicine and surgery. 3rd edition. St Louis (MO): WB Saunders; 2011. p. 451–71.
10. Nieminen P, Mustonen AM, Kärjä V, et al. Fatty acid composition and development of hepatic lipidosis during food deprivation–mustelids as a potential animal model for liver steatosis. Exp Biol Med 2009;234:278–86.
11. Antic V, Tempini A, Montani JP. Serial changes in cardiovascular and renal function of rabbits ingesting a high-fat, high-calorie diet. Am J Hypertens 1999;12:826–9.
12. Hsu HH, Culley NC. Effects of dietary calcium on atherosclerosis, aortic calcification, and icterus in rabbits fed a supplemental cholesterol diet. Lipids Health Dis 2006;5:16.
13. Clauss M, Burger B, Liesegang A, et al. Influence of diet on calcium metabolism, tissue calcification and urinary sludge in rabbits (*Oryctolagus cuniculus*). J Anim Physiol Anim Nutr 2012;96:798–807.
14. Harcourt-Brown F. Urinogenital diseases. Textbook of rabbit medicine. Oxford (United Kingdom): Butterworth Heinemann; 2002. p. 335–51.
15. Klaphake E, Paul-Murphy J. Disorders of the reproductive and urinary systems. In: Quesenberry KE, Carpenter JW, editors. Ferrets, rabbits and rodents: clinical medicine and surgery. 3rd edition. St Louis (MO): WB Saunders; 2011. p. 217–31.
16. Kamphues J. Calcium metabolism of rabbits as an etiological factor for urolithiasis. J Nutr 1991;121:S95–6.
17. Nyomba BL, Bouillon R, De Moor P. Influence of vitamin D status on insulin secretion and glucose tolerance in the rabbit. Endocrinology 1984;115:191–7.
18. Brommage R, Miller SC, Langman CB, et al. The effects of chronic vitamin D deficiency on the skeleton in the adult rabbit. Bone 1988;9:131–9.
19. White RN. Management of calcium ureterolithiasis in a French lop rabbit. J Small Anim Pract 2001;42:595–8.
20. Whary MT, Peper RL. Calcium carbonate urolithiasis in a rabbit. Lab Anim Sci 1994;44:534–6.
21. Harcourt-Brown FM. Diagnosis of renal disease in rabbits. Vet Clin North Am Exot Anim Pract 2013;16:145–74.
22. Gidenne T, Carabaño R, Garcia J, et al. Fibre digestion. In: de Blas C, Wiseman J, editors. The nutrition of the rabbit. Cambridge (MA): CABI; 2003. p. 69–88.
23. Lichtenberger M, Lennox AM. Emergency and critical care of small mammals. In: Quesenberry KE, Carpenter JW, editors. Ferrets, rabbits and rodents: clinical medicine and surgery. 3rd edition. St Louis (MO): WB Saunders; 2011. p. 531–44.
24. Grannis J. US rabbit industry profile. Fort Collins (CO): Centers for Epidemiology and Rabbit Health, Center for Emerging Issues; 2002.
25. Lowe JA. Pet rabbit feeding and nutrition. In: de Blas C, Wiseman J, editors. The nutrition of the rabbit. Cambridge (MA): CABI; 2003. p. 309–32.
26. Blas E, Gidenne T. Digestion of starch and sugars. In: de Blas C, Wiseman J, editors. The nutrition of the rabbit. Cambridge (MA): CABI; 2003. p. 17–38.

27. Lebas F, Gidenne T, Perez JM, et al. Nutrition and pathology. In: de Blas C, Wiseman J, editors. The nutrition of the rabbit. Cambridge (MA): CABI; 2003. p. 197–213.
28. Maertens L, Villamide MJ. Feeding systems for intensive production. In: de Blas C, Wiseman J, editors. The nutrition of the rabbit. Cambridge (MA): CABI; 2003. p. 255–72.
29. Njidda AA, Igwebuike JU. Growth performance and apparent nutrient digestibility of weanling rabbits fed graded levels of molasses. Global J Agr Sci 2007;6(1).
30. National Nutrient Database for Standard Reference: USDA, Agricultural Research Service, 2012. Available at: http://ndb.nal.usda.gov/ndb/foods. Accessed June 25, 2014.
31. Lawrence LM, Coleman RJ, Henning JC. Choosing hay for horses. Lexington (KY): University of Kentucky, Coop Ext Publ, Leaflet ID-146; 2000.

Supplements for Exotic Pets

Johanna Mejia-Fava, DVM, PhD[a],*,
Carmen M.H. Colitz, DVM, PhD, Diplomate ACVO[a,b]

KEYWORDS

- Alternative medicine • Supplements • Exotic pet • Herbal • Nutritional

KEY POINTS

- Animals have been choosing specific medicinal plants to treat their own diseases for as long as we can surmise. The practice of Zoopharmacognosy is discussed in detail showing that supplementation with plants has historically been documented in the wild.
- Dietary supplements are not as strictly regulated under the United States Food and Drug Administration (FDA) as prescription and over-the-counter drugs. Therefore, reputable nutraceutical companies should be committed to abiding by good manufacturing practices, choosing to work under accredited third-party certification providers.
- Vision, liver, immune, and stress supplement support are discussed because there is increasing scientific evidence of the effectiveness of these supplements in exotic species.
- It is increasingly important for the exotic animal practitioner to become knowledgeable about the various forms of complementary supplementation and research.

INTRODUCTION

This article discusses how practitioners can use nutritional and herbal supplements to support the health of exotic patients. Packaged Facts reported in 2013 that "a large share of non-dog/cat population are fish at 84.2 million, followed by birds at 11.4 million, reptiles at 3.9 million, followed by a range of other pets, including 5 million rabbits and hamsters."[1] Natural and organic pet foods, pet supplements, and other natural and organic pet supplies grew 5.2% in 2010 to reach $3.2 billion, with the animal supplement category adding $80 million in new sales to reach $1.6 billion.[2] If the most common diseases that affect exotic species are understood, then clinicians can try to prevent or alleviate disease states by providing supplements that both protect and support organ systems.

Disclosure: Dr J. Mejia-Fava is co-owner of Animal Necessity, LLC, a company that produces supplements for use in animals, some of which are discussed in this article.
[a] Animal Necessity, LLC, 45 West 34th Street, Suite 1107, New York, NY 10001, USA; [b] All Animal Eye Care, Inc., 300 South Central Boulevard, Jupiter, FL 33458, USA
* Corresponding author.
E-mail address: docjo@animal-necessity.com

Although it is accepted that food adaptations are critical to the survival of every species, it is not as readily apparent that food can also be purposefully used by animals for medicinal purposes. Zoopharmacognosy is the study of the ability of animals to recognize medicinal plants and other substances, and to ingest or otherwise apply them to their bodies to help prevent or treat disease.[3–5] Observations of animals healing themselves with natural medicinal foods have been recorded since ancient times.[3–5] Some herbs such as dog grass (*Agropyron repens*), catnip (*Nepeta cataria*), and horny goat weed (*Epimedium* spp) still carry the common names of the species using them medicinally. The term zoopharmacognosy was coined by Dr Eloy Rodriguez, a biochemist and professor at Cornell University.[5] This principle was popularized in 1987, when researchers investigated animals in the wild that were self-medicating by using the medicinal properties of plants, soils, clays, fungi, and insects.[5] Chimpanzees with diarrhea were confirmed to have intestinal parasitism with *Oesophagostomum stephanostomumto*.[5] Twenty hours after eating the pith of the *Vernonia* tree, one female's fecal excretion had lower levels of parasitism. Vernonioside B1, a compound isolated from the pith, was found to possess antiparasitic, antitumor, and antibacterial properties.[5] Other research shows that chimpanzees eat *Aspilia* leaves for their antiparasitic properties during the rainy season, because this is when parasitic larvae abound and there is increased risk of infection. The leaves are swallowed whole because they contain an oil called thiarubrine A, a compound that may decrease the ability of parasites to adhere to the intestinal wall.[4,5] The leaves also have unique Velcro-like hairs to which worms attach after passing through the digestive tract.[5] Humans use the *Aspilia* plant for a wide variety of diseases such as malaria, rheumatism, sciatica, and scurvy.[5] Other animals have used remedies for reproduction. African elephants seek a particular tree of the *Boraginaceae* family at the end of their gestation to induce labor.[5] The leaves and bark induce uterine contractions; pregnant Kenyan woman drink them in a tea to induce labor or abortion.[5] Fur rubbing has been observed in primates and bears that coat their fur with masticated plant materials as an insect repellant.[5] More than 200 species of songbird have a behavior called anting, in which they crush ants and rub them into their plumage. These crushed ants release formic acid, which is harmful to feather lice.[5]

Herbivorous and omnivorous mammals, birds, reptiles, and insects consume soil, stone, clay, and rock for medicinal purposes. The act of geophagy has been linked to alleviating diseases of the gastrointestinal tract (GIT).[3–5] Giraffes eat clay-rich termite mound soil for its detoxifying and absorptive properties. One clay mineral found in termite soil is kaolinite, which is the principal ingredient in the commercially available antidiarrheal drug, bismuth subsalicylate (Kaopectate).[5] Other reasons why animals use geophagy may be as a means to maintain proper gut pH, as a way to meet nutritional requirements, and to use sodium to detoxify secondary metabolites from consumed plants.[5] Dusky-footed wood rats have been observed to fumigate their nests by making tears in bay leaves, which release fumigating vapors that significantly reduce parasite survival.[5] Dogs commonly show plant-eating behaviors that are presumed to address a dietary deficiency of fiber, which has beneficial effects on energy metabolism, fecal characteristics, and digestive transit time.[6] The behavior of dogs eating grasses and then vomiting has been interpreted as both self-medication for gastrointestinal distress and as a form of relieving gas pressure in the stomach.[6] Cape foxes intentionally eat grass during periods of starvation to maintain digestive function.[6]

Another form of zoopharmacognosy is sponge carrying by Shark Bay dolphins of Australia. In one study, 5 sponge-carrying dolphins were found to be either solitary females, or females with dependent calves. All of these dolphins were healthy and reproduced successfully.[7] These sponges were surmised to be a natural marine product with antibacterial, antifungal, cytotoxic, and antimitotic properties.[7] Sponges contain spicules made of calcium carbonate, silica, and spongin (a natural type of collagen protein similar to keratin).[8] The study mentioned difficulty observing dolphins ingesting the sponges; perhaps the dolphins were not ingesting sponges but exploiting a compound in the sponges they carried.[7] During their prenatal and postnatal periods, sponge ingestion may have been a natural mechanism to achieve increased calcium levels in dolphins.

Zoopharmacognosy has enhanced clinicians' ability to better supplement exotic patients. Exotic animals under human care are blocked from using wild, natural dietary components. The exotic pet owner must therefore provide all of the nutrients that the animal needs, making knowledgeable dietary supplementation a cornerstone of lifetime wellness.

IS IT ALTERNATIVE MEDICINE OR TRADITIONAL/ORIGINAL MEDICINE?

Many private exotic specialty practices use at least one form of alternative medicine for their patients. However, the literature is lacking on the topic of supplement use in exotic species. Most of the current knowledge is extrapolated from human and small animal medicine. Therapeutic practices that incorporate supplements are described as holistic, integrative, and/or complementary and alternative medicine (CAM). The National Center for Complementary and Alternative Medicine[9] classifies CAM into different categories including mind-body medicine (acupuncture, meditation), body-based practices (chiropractic manipulation, massage), energy medicine (Reiki, therapeutic touch), whole medicine systems, and biologically based practices.[9,10]

As an exotic animal practitioner and also both a formulator and consumer of natural products, one of the authors (JMF) has extensive personal experience with the use of nutritional and herbal supplements. The author agrees that "...in order to authentically criticize (either positively or negatively) any 'alternative' modality, the practitioner must have tried it in a clinical environment and/or for personal use. This, of course, presupposes that the practitioner has versed him/herself in the modality with sufficient study to apply it in an appropriate manner."[11]

This article focuses on biologically based practices (nutritional and herbal supplements) used in exotic species (**Boxes 1–4**).

REGULATION

Dietary supplements are not as strictly regulated under the United States Food and Drug Administration (FDA) as prescription and over-the-counter drugs.[27] Under the Dietary Supplement Health and Education Act of 1994 (DSHEA), the manufacturer is responsible for ensuring that the supplement is safe before it goes to market.[27] Supplements are not considered a drug and therefore are not intended to treat, diagnose, mitigate, prevent, or cure diseases. Reputable nutraceutical companies committed to abiding by good manufacturing practices voluntarily choose to work under accredited third-party certification providers. These certification providers allow stakeholders (industry, regulators, users, and the general public) to determine compliance with regulatory specifications, correct label claims and packaging, and proper quantity and purity of ingredients. These providers include the National Animal Supplement Council, Natural Product Association, Natural Safety Foundation, Consumer-Lab, and US Pharmacopeial Convention. These certifications are not mandatory;

Box 1
Avian nutritional supplements and dosages

Agent	Dosage	Species
ALA	250 mg/kg of diet[12]	Japanese quail
Calcium	3–10 mg/kg feed (0.3–1%)[13]	Laying parrots
Essential fatty acids	0.5 mL/kg PO q 24 h × 50 d or indefinitely[13]	Raptors
Fatty acids (omega-3, omega-6)	0.1–0.2 mL/kg of flaxseed oil to corn oil mixed at a ratio of 1:4 PO or added to food; ratio of omega-6/omega-3 is 4–5:1[13]	Psittacines and pigeons
Fatty acids (omega-3, omega-6)	0.11 mL/kg q 24 h in a 5:1 ratio of omega-3[13]	Psittacines
Iodine (Lugol iodine)	0.2 mL/L drinking water daily[13]	Most bird species
	2 parts iodine + 28 parts water; 3 drops into 100 mL drinking water[13]	Budgerigars
Iodine (sodium iodide 20%)	2 mg (0.01 mL)/bird IM prn[13]	Budgerigars
	60 mg (0.3 mL)/kg IM[13]	Most bird species
Lactobacillus (Bene-Bac, Pet-Ag)	1 pinch/d/bird[13]	Psittacines
	1 tsp/L hand-feeding formula[13]	Most bird species
Pancreatic enzyme powder (Viokase-V Powder, Fort Dodge)	2–5 g/kg[13]	Most bird species
	1/8 tsp/kg feed[13]	Most bird species
	1/8 tsp/60–120 g lightly oil-coated seed[13]	Most bird species
Vitamin A (Aquasol A Parenteral, Astra)	5000 IU/kg IM q24h × 14 days, then 250–1000 IU/kg q 24h PO[13]	Psittacines
Vitamin B₁ (thiamine)	1–2 mg/kg PO q 24 h[13]	Raptors, penguins, cranes
	25–30 mg/kg fish (wet basis)[13]	Piscivorous species
Vitamin B₁₂ (cyanocobalamin)	0.25–0.5 mg/kg IM q 7 d[13]	Most bird species
	2–5 mg/bird SC[13]	Pigeons
Vitamin C (ascorbic acid)	20–50 mg/kg IM q 1–7 d[13]	Most bird species
	150 mg/kg PO q 24 h[13]	Willow ptarmigan chicks
Vitamin D₃ (Vital E-A + D, Schering)	3300 IU/kg (1000 U/300 g) IM q7d prn[13]	Most bird species
	6600 IU/kg IM once[13]	Most bird species
Vitamin E (Vitamin E20, Horse Health Products; Bo-SE, Schering Plough)	0.06 mg/kg IM q 7 d[13]	Psittacines
Vitamin E/γ- linolenic acid (2%), linoleic acid (71%)(Derm Caps, DVM Pharmaceuticals)	0.1 mL/kg PO q 24 h[13]	Most bird species
	4000 mg linolenic acid/kg feed[13]	Japanese quail
Policosanol	0.3–2.0 mg/kg orally[14]	Most bird species
Melissa or lemon balm (*Melissa officinalis*)	Topically applied for irritated papillomatous lesions with sterile lubrication jelly with enough volume to contact the papilloma surface[15]	Most bird species
Yarrow (*Achillea millefolium*)	Topically used for slow-healing wounds and skin inflammation as well as clotting in oozing wounds[15]	Most bird species
Eye Sea	Screech owls: average weight: 208 g (0.2 kg [0.44 lb]) Dilute 1 capsule into 10 mL of water, then make into 0.5-mL aliquots for 20 animals Dose: give one-twentieth of a capsule per 0.2–1.36 kg[16]	Screech owls, unpublished data

(continued on next page)

Box 1 (continued)		
Agent	**Dosage**	**Species**
OcuGlo (small bottle)	1 capsule orally for animals less than 4.5 kg (10 lb)[17]	Chinese goose
Imuno-2865	1000 mg SID for estimated weight (3 kg)[18]	Penguins
Shana-Vet	500 mg SID for estimated weight (3 kg)[18]	Penguins

Abbreviations: ALA, alpha lipoic acid; IM, intramuscular; PO, orally; prn, as needed; q, every; SC, subcutaneously; SID, single intradermal dose; tsp, teaspoon.

companies that hold these seals of approval proactively provide the best quality supplements to their consumers, and veterinarians should responsibly seek out these products. A recent study found that 34 of 44 herbal products tested were contaminated with some type of substitution or filler, which poses serious health risks to consumers.[28] This study shows the importance of finding a company that is certified at executing good manufacturing practices (GMPs) for pharmaceutical grade and not food-grade standards. GMP refers to the regulations promulgated by the FDA under the authority of the Federal Food, Drug, and Cosmetic Act. Failure of GMP-certified firms to comply with GMP regulations can result in serious consequences including recall fines and incarceration. GMP regulations address issues including record keeping, personnel qualifications, sanitation, cleanliness, equipment verification, process validation, and complaint handling.[27] Manufacturers that do not comply with GMP standards should not be recommended.

Box 2 Ferrets, rabbits, guinea pigs, and rodent nutritional supplements and dosages		
Agent	**Dosage**	**Species**
Ferrets		
Nutri-Cal (EVSCO)	1–3 mL/animal PO q 6–8 h[13]	Ferrets
Saw palmetto	0.15 mL/animal PO q 12 h[13]	Ferrets
Yeast, brewer's	1/8–1/4 tsp PO q 12 h[13]	Ferrets
Rabbits		
Lactobacilli	Administer PO during antibiotic treatment period, then 5–7 d beyond cessation[13]	Rabbits
Silymarin	4–15 mg/kg PO q 8–12 h[13]	Rabbits
(milk thistle)	20–50 mg/kg PO q 24 h[13]	Rabbits
Hedgehogs		
Lactobacilli	2.5 mL/kg q 24 h[13]	Hedgehogs
Rodents		
Vitamin C (ascorbic acid)	50–100 mg/kg PO, SC, IM q 24 h[13]	Guinea pigs
Lactobacilli	PO during antibiotic treatment period, then 5–7 d beyond cessation; give 2 h before or 2 h following antibiotic treatment[13]	All rodent species
Echinacea	2 mg/mouse/d[15]	Mice
Milk thistle (*Silybum marianum*)	4–15 mg/kg PO q 8–12 h[13]	Most rodent species

Box 3
Reptiles, fish, cetaceans, and primate nutritional supplements and dosages

Reptiles

Iron dextran	12 mg/kg IM 1–2 × wk × 45 d[13]	Crocodilians/iron deficiency; in other species for anemia[96]
Vitamin A	1000–5000 U/kg IM q 7–10 d × 4 treatments[13]	Most reptile species
	2000 U/kg PO, SC, IM q 7–14 d × 2–4 treatments[13]	Most reptile species
Vitamins A, D_3, E (Vital E+A+D, Stuart Products)	0.15 mL/kg IM, repeat in 21 d[13]	Most reptile species
	0.3 mL/kg PO, then 0.06 mL/kg q 7 d × 3–4 treatments[13]	Box turtles
Vitamin B complex	0.3 mL/kg SC, IM q 24 h[13]	Most reptile species
	25 mg thiamine/kg PO q 24 h × 3–7 d[13]	Most reptile species
Vitamin B_1 (thiamin)	50–100 mg/kg PO, SC, IM q 24 h[13]	Piscivores
	30 g/kg feed fish PO[13]	Crocodilians
Vitamin B_{12} (cyanocobalamin)	0.05 mg/kg SC, IM q 24 h[13]	Snakes, lizards
Vitamin C	10–20 mg/kg SC, IM[13]	All reptile species
Vitamin D_3	1000 IU/kg IM, repeat in 1 wk[13]	Most reptile species
Vitamin E/selenium (L-Se, Schering)	1 IU vitamin E/kg IM[13]	Piscivores
	50 IU vitamin E/kg + 0.025 mg selenium/kg IM[13]	Lizards
Vitamin K_1	0.25–0.5 mg/kg IM[13]	Most reptile species
Carnitine	250 mg/kg[19]	All reptile species
Methionine	40–50 mg/kg[19]	Dose seems safe in most reptiles
Milk thistle (*Silybum marianum*)	4–15 mg/kg PO q 8–12 h[13]	Lizards
Omega-3	600 mg SID at 27 kg[20]	Atlantic Ridley sea turtle
Lecithin	1200 mg SID at 27 kg[20]	Atlantic Ridley sea turtle
Alpha lipoic acid	100 mg SID at 27 kg[20]	Atlantic Ridley sea turtle
Artichoke and milk thistle	1650 mg SID at 27 kg[20]	Atlantic Ridley sea turtle

Fish

Iodine derivative	10–30 mg kg body weight-1 week-1[21]	Elasmobranchs: this dosage is recommended in facilities where goiter is expected to develop. This dosage is more than a dietary supplement and may be high for some species

Cetaceans

Imuno-2865	5–15 mg/kg[22,23]	Atlantic bottlenose dolphin
Serenin Vet	Follow Animal Necessity dosing guidelines by weight[24]	Atlantic bottlenose dolphin
Shana Vet	Follow Animal Necessity dosing guidelines by weight. Topical form should be applied after drying the area as the cream is water resistant[24]	Atlantic bottlenose dolphin
Alpha lipoic acid	2–3 mg/kg[25]	California sea lion

Primates

Tryptophan	Tryptophan supplementation at 100 mg/kg q 24 h in the afternoon reduced self-mutilation[26]	Rhesus monkey

> **Box 4**
> **Veterinary supplement resources**
>
> - National Center for Complementary and Alternative Medicine (NCCAM): http://nccam. nih.gov/
> - American Holistic Veterinary Medical Association (AHVMA): http://www.ahvma.org/
> - Veterinary Botanical Medical Association (VBMA): http://www.vbma.org/
> - Natural Standard: http://www.naturalstandard.com/
> - National Animal Supplement Council (NASC): http://www.nasc.cc/
> - Animal Necessity, LLC: http://animal-necessity.com
> - Oxbow Animal Health: http://www.oxbowanimalhealth.com/
> - Harrison's Bird Foods: http://www.harrisonsbirdfoods.com/products/avix.html
> - Lafeber: http://lafeber.com

VITAMIN AND MINERALS
Vitamin A

Vitamin A is composed of the fat-soluble retinoids, including retinol, retinal, retinoic acid, and retinyl esters.[29] Preformed vitamin A (retinol and its esterified form, retinyl ester) and provitamin A carotenoids (beta carotene, alpha carotene, and beta cryptoxanthin) are two forms commonly found in food.[29] Both of these forms of vitamin A are converted into retinol, then oxidized first to retinal, and then to retinoic acid.[29] Vitamin A is stored in the liver as retinyl esters. Retail supplements on the market that contain vitamin A are usually found in forms of animal-based retinol esters (palmitate, acetate) or plant-based precursors (beta carotene). Careful attention is advised as to which type of vitamin A is administered to exotic patients. The smaller the animal, the less room for error, and the greater the chance of toxicity because this is a fat-soluble vitamin that, in excess, is stored in adipocytes.[30] Retinyl palmitate is a more stable version of retinol, but skin must further break down retinyl palmitate, therefore much higher concentrations are required to provide the similar benefit.[31,32] Two molecules of vitamin A are formed from 1 molecule of beta carotene. The body converts beta carotene into retinol in the amount needed, which makes this a safer form of vitamin A.[31,32]

Herbivores, such as green sea turtles, feed on seagrass and convert beta carotene to vitamin A.[33] Carnivores and many turtles, such as the box turtle, are less capable of converting beta carotene to vitamin A.[33] These animals require an animal-based retinol ester in their diets.[33] In order to provide adequate vitamin A, a high-quality diet should be provided, including dark leafy greens and orange and yellow vegetables. Birds on an all-seed diet should be changed to a commercial high-quality pelleted feed that is always well within its expiration date. Insectivores should ingest insects that are fed, or gut-loaded with, vegetables. In addition, the insects should be dusted weekly with a multivitamin containing preformed vitamin A.[33]

Vitamin C

Deficiencies in vitamin C and zinc may result in abnormal cartilage development and maintenance.[34] Sandtiger sharks (*Carcharias taurus*) in captivity have been reported to have spinal deformities related to a nutritional deficiency of vitamin C, vitamin E, and zinc.[34] In exotic pets, hypovitaminosis C (scurvy) is commonly seen in the guinea pig. Owners should feed commercial guinea pig pellets containing fortified levels of vitamin C that exceed maintenance requirements. Approximately one-half of vitamin C is oxidized and inactivated within 90 days in fortified diets. Dampness, heat, and light can reduce the level of vitamin C, so pet owners should be aware of expiration dates both on diets and supplement bottles. Some clinical signs include poor fur coat quality, swollen knee joints, lameness, gingival bleeding, chronic nonhealing skin wounds, and diarrhea.[33] Maintenance vitamin C requirements for guinea pigs are 10 mg/kg body weight daily, 30 mg/kg body weight for pregnant animals, and higher doses (50 mg/kg) may be suggested for sick or convalescent animals.[33] Hypervitaminosis C has been reported in guinea pigs, so careful and accurate dosing when supplementing should be monitored.[35] Vitamin C also increases absorption of iron so caution must be exercised in animals prone to hemachromatosis or if there is iron supplementation.

Vitamin D, Calcium, and Phosphorus

Unlike other mammals, rabbits absorb calcium readily from the GIT without vitamin D or activation of calcium-binding proteins within the GIT. Owners must not oversupplement rabbits with vitamin D because hypercalcemia can occur. Many modern species, including amphibians, reptiles, birds, and most mammals, still depend on sunlight for their vitamin D requirements.[36,37] Avian skin covered with plumage cannot synthesize vitamin D. Nonfeathered skin, including the legs, has a 10-fold higher concentration of 7-dehydrocholesterol.[36,37] Cats have no 7-dehyrocholesterol in their skins and therefore cannot synthesize vitamin D_3. They depend solely on diet for their vitamin D_3 requirement.[35,36]

Commercial supplements are available with and without vitamin D_3. A supplement that contains vitamin D_3 and not vitamin D_2 is recommended. Vitamin D_2 has not been shown to support normal skeletal mineralization in amphibians.[35,36] The author recommends that if an exotic pet is exposed to natural sunlight or full-spectrum lighting (ultraviolet B range, 285–320 nm), then caution should be taken to avoid oversupplementation with vitamin D_3.[38] Vitamin D_3 is fat soluble, which can induce toxicity, and, in excess, is stored in adipocytes.

Supplemental calcium can be provided by dusting food with pure calcium carbonate, calcium citrate, or calcium lactate. Calcium gluconate is also acceptable and can be compounded as a liquid for oral administration. Pure calcium that is free of heavy metals, such as lead, should be used to make sure there is no interference with normal metabolism. Calcium sources include oyster shell, cuttle bone, ground calcium carbonate tablets, and gut loading insects with calcium. Pelleted diets are important for psittacines to avoid deleterious self-selection of calcium-deficient seeds.

Deficiency of vitamin D has been linked to immunosuppression and autoimmune disease.[39] Vitamin D receptors are present in tissues involved in calcium homeostasis and also in tissues associated with immunomodulation.[39] In addition, vitamin D possesses antiinflammatory properties such as augmenting macrophage function and the inhibition of inflammatory cytokines such as tumor necrosis factor alpha and interleukins.[39] The author (JMF) found that vitamin D levels in wild-caught, whole frozen capelin, smelt, and squid were negligible (JMF, unpublished data, 2014). Therefore, when feeding carnivorous aquatic species housed indoors, it is prudent to supplement with Vitamin D.

Thiamine and Vitamin E

Thiaminase in the meat of certain fish species is not destroyed by the freezing process and, over time, especially in poorly stored fish, continues to break down thiamine.[40–43] If animals are not supplemented with thiamine, neurotoxicity can occur, and manifests as ataxia, muscle tremors, blindness, and even death.[40–43]

Vitamin E deficiency causes anorexia and painful swollen subcutaneous nodules. Steatitis has been reported in reptiles such as crocodiles and sea turtles, as well as in birds, mammals, and fish.[44] Marine and cold-water fish store energy as polyunsaturated fats, which in the presence of oxygen induce peroxidation and rancidity, which in turn depletes vitamin E levels.[45] Fish-eating animals should be fed wholesome, fresh fish that are fresh frozen and thawed in cool temperatures.[44]

Vitamin E is an important antioxidant that protects unsaturated lipids from degradation by reactive oxygen species.[46] The quantity of unsaturated fatty acids in tissues dictates the vitamin E requirement.[46] The author (JMF) found that vitamin E levels in wild-caught, whole frozen Atlantic herring, capelin, and smelt were negligible.[47] Aquatic mammal, avian, fish, and reptile species on carnivorous diets need vitamin E supplementation because of the high proportion of dietary unsaturated fatty acids. Excessive concentrations of vitamin E may inhibit vitamin C absorption.[34] Vitamin E should be provided in combination with another antioxidant such as vitamin C or grape-seed extract (GSE), which reduce tocopheroxyl radicals back to their active state.[48,49] In addition, GSE is a more potent free radical scavenger than vitamins C and E.[50]

Iodine

Iodine deficiency can be caused by lack of dietary intake, iodine-deficient soils, and dietary goitrogens. Goiter has been reported in giant terrestrial tortoises (*Geochelone elephantopus* and *Testudo gigantea*) as well as budgerigars when fed goitrogenic vegetables.[51,52] Vegetables high in goitrogens should be fed only intermittently; these include kale, bok choy, turnips, cabbage, broccoli, and cauliflower.

Iodine is also essential for fish and dietary requirements are still unknown. Diffusion uptake of iodide occurs across the gills and stomach, with excretion primarily in the kidneys and rectal gland.[21] A disinfectant, such as ozone, causes a reduction of iodide.[53] Normal iodine uptake can also be inhibited by increased levels of bromide, fluoride, calcium, cobalt, manganese, and sulfides.[21]

Herring, capelin, and smelt are fish that are commonly fed to aquatic species. In 1989, Lall[54] reported that substantial losses of iodine occur during processing of fish meal. Levels of iodine measured in 3 types of fishmeal were low (ie, 5–10 mg per kg).[54] The author (JMF) found that iodine, selenium, and vitamin C levels in these fish, when frozen, are negligible.[47] Vitamin C deficiency can also reduce iodide uptake.[21] Selenium deficiency has been associated with a form of hypothyroidism.[44] Although this type of Se-deficiency hypothyroidism has only been described in mammals, it should also be suspected in reptiles fed foods from selenium-deficient regions as well as aquatic species fed frozen-fish diets.[44]

Because safe levels of iodine have not been reported for many exotic species, caution should be exercised with iodine supplementation. Nutritional requirements for iodine depend on age, growth, sex, physiologic status, environmental stress, disease, reproductive stage, lactation, and iodine content in the water.[54] To meet daily requirements, humans must trap 60 μg of dietary iodine; daily recommendations for growth are 50 to 150 μg; for reproduction 175 to 200 μg; and lactation 290 μg.[44] Because reptiles have a lower metabolic rate than humans, an adequate daily level is approximately one-fourth to one-third of human levels (0.3 g/kg body weight).[44] Iodine can be supplemented as iodized salt (potassium iodide, sodium iodide, or calcium iodate) or algae (seaweeds) in powder and tablet forms.[21] There are several macroalgae, such as *Spirulina* and *Chlorella vulgaris*, in which it has been determined that iodine content depends on the method of algae cultivation.[55,56] Other algae such as dried kelp contain an average iodine content of 0.062% to 620 μg/g, which is about 8 times the iodine content of iodized salt.[44] The kelp industry is well regulated in Norway and Japan, but not all kelp products sold in the United States are regulated.[44] Because iodine content of algae can vary, the authors recommend contacting the company from which algae is purchased to determine the concentration and source of iodine.

SUPPLEMENTAL SUPPORT
Specific Antioxidants with Beneficial Ocular Effects

Carotenoids include lutein, zeaxanthin, and lycopene. Lutein and zeaxanthin are oxycarotenoids found in dark leafy vegetables, egg yolks, and colored fruits. They selectively accumulate in the lens and the retina; they are also found in the uveal tract with trace amounts found in the cornea and sclera.[57,58] Lutein and zeaxanthin may be particularly effective in the prevention or slowing of cataract; increased plasma and/or dietary levels of these carotenoids are associated with decreased risk of cataract formation. Animals fed diets lacking lutein and zeaxanthin were more susceptible to cataract development. Lutein and zeaxanthin also have protective effects on the retina against blue light and oxidative stress.[59] Together with the metabolite mesozeaxanthin, they accumulate in photoreceptor axons and interneurons of the inner plexiform layer.[60] Lutein exists primarily in the rod photoreceptor outer segments.[61] In birds, lutein and zeaxanthin accumulate in the retina, specifically in the cone-rich retina, where they exist as esters in oil droplets.[62] Dietary lutein was detectable in the blood and retinas of supplemented marine mammals and green sea turtles.[63,64] Lutein also has antiinflammatory effects via the nuclear factor kappa B pathway.[65] Lycopene is found primarily in tomatoes and has the highest physical quenching rate constant with singlet oxygen species compared with all other known carotenoids. Lycopene has been shown to protect against cataract formation in vitro and in animal models.[66]

Flavonoids are also phytochemicals with antioxidant and antiinflammatory properties. Flavonoids are found in bilberry, GSE, green tea extract, and quercetin. Bilberry and GSE inhibit oxidative stress and GSE has been shown to inhibit formation of certain types of cataracts in animal models by increasing glutathione, the predominant antioxidant system in the lens.[67] Epigallocatechin gallate (EGCG), the principal flavonoid in green tea, may be a beneficial complement to glaucoma therapy because it protects against ischemia/reperfusion injury[68] and seems to have neuroprotective effects on the inner retina.[69,70] EGCG also protects photoreceptors in models of oxidative stress–induced retinal degeneration.[71] Green tea catechins have been detected in the retina and aqueous humor after oral administration. Similar to other plant extracts, green tea has many constituents and all have some effective antioxidant capabilities; therefore their combination provides free radical scavenging effects, antioxidant effects, and lipid peroxidation inhibition.[72] Green tea extracts likely convey protective effects against cataract formation, as has been shown in an animal model of selenite-induced cataracts.[73] Quercetin reaches measurable plasma levels when provided in meals rich in various fruits and vegetables.[74] Following uptake into the lens, quercetin is metabolized to 3'-O-methyl quercetin, which is also protective against oxidative stress.[75] Therefore, quercetin may have protective effects against cataract formation.

Omega fatty acids (OFA) of the n-3 and n-6 series are important components of cell membrane phospholipids and cannot be interconverted.[76] Docosahexaenoic acid (DHA) and eicosapentaenoic acid (EPA), commonly termed omega-3 fatty acids, are found in fish and other marine animals because they are synthesized at the base of the aquatic food chain by phytoplankton. Omega-3 fatty acids are also found in flaxseed, pumpkin seeds, and green leafy vegetables. Preformed dietary polyunsaturated fatty acids, such as fish oils, are a more efficient way to supplement diets with DHA than flaxseed oil. DHA is present in high levels in the retina, cerebral cortex, sperm, and testis,[77] and is found in the photoreceptor outer segments. Together with lutein and zeaxanthin, DHA promotes photoreceptor health and protection against oxidative stress.[78]

Alpha lipoic acid (ALA) is a cofactor for alpha-keto-dehydrogenase complexes, participating in acyl transfer reactions.[79] ALA and its reduced form, dihydrolipoic acid, have potent antioxidant abilities.[80] ALA is normally found in small amounts in mammalian tissues bound to enzyme complexes. This bound form is unavailable to function as an antioxidant. However, free exogenous ALA may be an effective thiol substitute.[81] ALA has been shown to protect against cataract formation and showed increases in ascorbate, vitamin E, and glutathione.[82]

By supplementing a variety of antioxidant nutraceuticals, endogenous and exogenous eye diseases may benefit. A mouse model of inherited retinal degeneration had increased antioxidant levels, reduced photoreceptor cell death, and reduced oxidatively damaged DNA when supplemented with lutein, zeaxanthin, ALA, and *Lycium barbarum* extract.[83] A commercially available antioxidant blend was safely used in a Chinese goose with cataracts for more than a year, and the cataracts remained stable.[17] A similar nutraceutical blend has also been used safely in screech owls in a recent toxicity study.[16] It is the authors' opinion that a variety of antioxidants is ideal as a complement to an appropriate diet.

LIVER SUPPORT

Hepatic lipidosis (excessive lipid accumulation in hepatocytes) is a metabolic derangement caused by multiple factors linked to diet, obesity, reduced activity, and seasonal vitellogenesis in reptile, avian, and aquatic species.[19,20,84,85] Methionine, biotin, and choline are essential nutrients for humans and animals and a deficiency may inhibit formation of lipoproteins, thereby inhibiting mobilization of fat and resulting in hepatic lipidosis. This condition is commonly seen in psittaciforme species such as budgerigars, cockatiels, Amazon parrots, and cockatoos.[86] Treatment entails correcting dietary or environmental factors, addressing concurrent disease, and supporting liver regeneration. In birds, the level of protein should be decreased to approximately 8%, vitamin A reduced to 1500 IU/kg of diet, and branched chain amino acids (leucine, isoleucine, and valine) should be increased in a ratio of 2:1 to aromatic amino acids.[87] Ahlstrom and colleagues reported the beneficial use of nutraceuticals for a case of hepatic lipidosis in an Atlantic Ridley sea turtle (*Lepidocheyls kempii*).[20] The supplementation protocol for this animal included artichoke and milk thistle, ALA, lecithin, and omega-3 fatty acids; these resulted in dramatic improvements in serum biochemistry liver values as well as behavior, characterized by normal diving and swimming activity.[20]

ALA

ALA is a naturally occurring dithiol compound that is an essential cofactor for mitochondrial bioenergetics enzymes.[87] ALA recycles glutathione, which is considered the universal antioxidant found in highest concentrations in the brain, eye, heart, and liver.[88,89] Glutathione is a nutrient formed from 3 amino acids, 2 of which are the essential amino acids cysteine and methionine. Glutathione levels can become depleted when there is a heavy toxicity load in the liver, allowing toxins to build up in the body. Glutathione is needed by the liver in order to change fat-soluble toxins into water-soluble toxins, which are then excreted by the kidneys.[88] ALA has been studied in Japanese quail to ameliorate undesired lipid peroxidation effects caused by heat stress as well as preventive effects of atherosclerosis.[12,90] The maximum tolerated dose for cats is 13 mg/kg body weight, which is significantly lower than the single oral dose tolerated in humans, dogs, and rats: 120, 126, and 635 mg/kg, respectively.[89] Further research needs to be performed to assess safe doses for exotic species. ALA also recycles vitamin C (ascorbic acid) and has diverse antioxidant and pharmacologic properties including improving glycemic control, directly terminating free radicals, and chelating transition metal ions including iron and copper.[80] ALA decreases blood glucose levels, therefore animals that are diabetic and being administered insulin or with low blood glucose levels should be monitored carefully.

S-adenosy-L-methionine

S-adenosy-L-methionine (SAMe) also increases glutathione levels using a different mechanism. SAMe donates its methyl group to choline transforming into S-adeno-syl-homocysteine (SAH). Homocysteine is normally converted to SAMe, which recycles back to methionine or, alternatively, is converted to cysteine and then to glutathione. Vitamin B_6, B_{12}, and folic acid (SAMe's main cofactors) are essential for the recycling of homocysteine.[91] If these B vitamins are deficient in the diet, SAMe may not break down properly and homocysteine levels may accumulate to unsafe levels.

SAMe plays a role in more than 100 reactions catalyzed by methyltransferases. These reactions include biosynthesis of creatine; formation of neurotransmitters and some neuroreceptors; biosynthesis of phospholipids; biosynthesis of L-carnitine; and reactions involving DNA, RNA, and proteins.[92] Hepatic SAMe serves as the major source of hepatic glutathione and systemic thiol. Increased blood homocysteine levels are a risk factor for atherothrombotic vascular disease and other cardiac diseases.[93]

Lecithin, Inositol, Phosphatidylcholine, and Methionine

Lecithin, inositol, and phosphatidylcholine (PC) are in a class of phospholipids that incorporate choline as a headgroup. Choline is lipotropic, acting on fat metabolism by hastening removal and converting fats into phospholipids, which are more rapidly transferred from the liver into blood.[19] The most likely toxic change of fatty liver disease is damage to the mitochondrial membranes causing inability of the liver parenchymal cells to metabolize fats.[94] PC is important in the known mechanisms of liver homeostasis, toxic liver damage, and the liver's recovery processes.[94] PC is a safer means of dietary choline repletion than choline itself.[94] Methionine is also a precursor to choline with reported lipotropic effects.[19]

Omega-3 Fatty Acids

Omega-3 fatty acids have several beneficial properties and supplementation has been used in various exotic pet species for hepatic lipidosis. One study evaluated 10 European polecats (*Mustela putorius*), the wild form of the domestic ferret, in which food was withheld for 5 days with 10 control animals fed a commercial diet.[95] The food-deprived animals showed microvesicular and macrovesicular hepatic steatosis. The most important biochemical manifestations shared by the polecats and humans with nonalcoholic fatty liver disease (NAFLD) were decreased total n-3 PUFA percentage and an increase in the n-6/n-3 PUFA ratio in liver and white adipose tissue.[95] Various mechanisms have been described through which consumption of fish oil has been beneficial in the alleviation of NAFLD, such as (1) decreased plasma nonesterified fatty acid concentrations; (2) decreased de novo lipogenesis, very-low-density lipoprotein export, and plasma triglyceride concentrations; and (iii) decreased adipocyte size and visceral fat content.[96]

Artichoke, Milk Thistle, and Dandelion

Concomitant intake of plant extracts containing cytoprotective compounds may increase the efficacy of treating liver disease. Artichoke, milk thistle, and dandelion have antioxidant liver protectant properties. Dandelion is a common plant fed to herbivorous reptile species. These supplements have been shown to have few side effects, although artichoke and dandelion do have diuretic properties and should be used with caution in dehydrated patients.

Artichoke (Cynara scolymus) is a flower extract that contains cynarin, a compound that promotes production of bile. Artichoke leaves contain caffeoylquinic acids, which help to improve digestion and aid in liver, gallbladder, and diuretic kidney function. This plant is used for medicinal purposes; it not only has hepatoprotective action but also prevents atherosclerosis and hyperlipidemia or dyspeptic disorders.[97]

Milk thistle (Silybum ebumeum or Silybum marianum) is a waxy-lobed, thorny plant that is a member of the daisy family. Milk thistle contains 80% silymarin, an important compound that nourishes the liver, helps protect it from cellular damage, and upregulates the antioxidant enzymes superoxide dismutase, catalase, glutathione peroxidase, glutathione reductase, and glutathione S-transferase.[98] Hepatoprotective effects against mushroom poisoning have been reported with silybin, the active ingredient of silymarin.[98] Pigeons were infected with aflatoxin after a 21-day period of milk thistle supplementation and results showed that there was a reduction in bile acid levels and white blood cell counts compared with nonsupplemented control animals.[98] Further studies are warranted to evaluate the hepatoprotectant effects of this supplement in avian species. Anecdotal accounts from bird owners report that they observe improved appetites in their animals after being supplemented with milk thistle.

Dandelion (Taraxacum officinale) has a wide array of therapeutic functions including choleretic, diuretic, antioxidant, antiinflammatory, and hepatoprotective properties.[99] A few studies have been performed evaluating the hepatoprotectant effects of dandelion in mice. Results in one study showed hepatoprotective effects after acetaminophen hepatotoxicity with a possible mechanism involving its free radical scavenger activities. This effect was attributed to the extract's content of phenolic compounds.[99] Another study used a murine model of methionine-deficient and choline-deficient diet, which induced nonalcoholic steatohepatitis (NASH). Results suggested that dandelion leaf extract has beneficial effects on NASH, mainly because of its antioxidant and antiinflammatory activities.[100]

IMMUNE, ANTIFUNGAL, ANTIVIRAL, ANTIINFLAMMATORY SUPPORT

In recent years, advances in testing of the different facets of exotic species' immune systems have resulted in a increase of knowledge, and research continues to expand this understanding. Pilot studies evaluated immune function using Imuno-2865 (PDS-2865) in cetacean species.[22,23] This new supplement is a beta-glucan that shows encouraging findings in improving human lymphocyte activation and interleukin activity.[101–103] Beta-glucans are polysaccharides with immune-modulating properties and are found in the bran of cereal grains; the cell wall of baker's yeast; and certain types of fungi, mushrooms, algae, and plants including members of the Poaceae (or Gramineae) family.[101–103] Various beta-glucan supplements are commercially available.

Arabinogalactan is found in various plants, with the highest concentrations occurring in larch trees. This starchlike chemical enhances beneficial gut microflora by increasing short-chain fatty acid production (primarily butyrate), which is both essential for proper immune health of the colon and is the preferred substrate for energy generation by colonic epithelial cells.[104] The effectiveness of beta-glucans is enhanced when delivered in small particle sizes (microparticulates) to help promote improved absorption and function in the immune system.[101–103] The laboratory extraction process used to break down or predigest beta-glucan polysaccharide molecules into smaller components, called hemicelluloses, makes them an ideal food supplement to support and enhance immune system function.

Eicosanoids are derived from omega-3 and omega-6 fatty acids. Omega-6 eicosanoids (gamma-linolenic and arachidonic acid [AA]) are proinflammatory, whereas omega-3 fatty acids (EPA and DHA) have antiinflammatory properties and may serve as potential therapeutic agents for cancer prevention and control.[105] In animal models, an increased ratio of dietary n-3 to n-6 fatty acids has been shown to inhibit the development of mammary cancer.[105] Omega-3 fatty acids exert their antiinflammatory effects in skin by acting as natural 5-lipooxygenase inhibitors of AA, as well as having antileukotriene and antineutrophilic properties.[106]

Common fungal organisms often invade the epidermis, keratin layer, and respiratory tract of various exotic species. Aspergillosis is a significant avian disease that can be challenging to diagnose. Prophylactic treatment with itraconazole in penguins is a common practice, in order to reduce morbidity and mortality, especially during periods of transport stress.[18] However, chronic use of itraconazole can promote antifungal drug resistance. A recent pilot study was therefore conducted to investigate whether an alternative prophylaxis using supplements (squalene, calendula, triacontanol, and beta-glucans) would have less adverse effects.[18] During a potentially stressful exhibit modification period, penguins were evaluated before and after supplementation using complete blood count, protein electrophoresis, *Aspergillus* antibody testing, and galactomannan antigen testing. Prophylactic supplementation of Shana-Vet and Imuno-2865 (PDS-2865) was used safely in 25 penguins and none of the birds developed fungal disease.[18]

Squalene is a natural lipid triterpene and is also a vital precursor of cholesterol biosynthesis.[107] Squalene is synthesized in humans, sharks, and other species.[107] Because of its significant dietary benefits, biocompatibility, and other advantageous properties, squalene is extensively used as an emollient and for photoprotection of skin in pharmaceutical formulations, and is used synergistically to enhance the cytocidal effect of antifungals.[107] High intracellular fungal squalene concentrations are thought to interfere with fungal membrane function and cell wall synthesis.[107] *Calendula* is a flower that contains sesquiterpenes, glycosides, saponins, xanthophylls, triol triterpenes, and flavonoids that have antiinflammatory effects.[108] This plant has been found to possess antifungal activity against 22 strains of pathogenic *Candida* species.[108] A major threat to agriculture and to human health is *Aspergillus flavus*, a common filamentous fungus that produces aflatoxins.[109] In the *A flavus* life cycle, the transition from sclerotia to conidia life-forms is governed by both lipoxygenase activity and cell density.[109] When exposed to *Aspergillus fumingatus*, *Candida albicans*, or *Cryptococcus neoformans*, alveolar macrophages may promote peroxidation of surfactant lipids in the lungs.[110] Found in high concentrations in beeswax and plant cuticle waxes, triacontanol is a 30-carbon alcohol that inhibits lipoxygenase.[111] Triacontanol has antiinflammatory effects that may be mediated through inhibition of lipid peroxidation.[111,112] Results of a study using a guinea pig skin model suggest that triacontanol-containing mixtures represent an alternative treatment modality to topical steroid applications.[111]

In addition to its antiinflammatory effects, triacontanol and docosanol show antiherpetic properties.[111,112] Docosanol, also known as behenyl alcohol, is a saturated 22-carbon aliphatic alcohol. Docosanol inhibits fusion between envelope viruses and host cells, thus blocking viral entry and replication.[113]

Aloe vera (L.) Burm. f. is a perennial succulent xerophyte found in various supplements.[114] The medicinal effects of this plant are attributed to polysaccharides found in the parenchyma of the inner leaves.[114] Therapeutic effects include antiinflammatory, laxative, immunostimulating, antibacterial, wound and burn healing, antiulcer of the GIT, antitumor, and antidiabetic activities.[114]

Shana-Vet contains calendula, triacontanol, docosanol, aloe vera, and squalene. Further research using this supplement (both topical and oral forms) is suggested in animals with herpesvirus. Oxbow Natural Science Skin & Coat contains chamomile, canola, and red palm oil, which provide antioxidant and antipruritic properties for skin-related diseases. Harrison's Booster and Sunshine Factor also contains red palm oil which is composed of approximately 50% saturated and 50% unsaturated fatty acids.[115] This antioxidant-rich oil also has significant concentrations of carotenoids and vitamin E (75% in the form of tocotrienol).[115] The oil has cardioprotective and antineoplastic properties.[115,116] Oxbow Natural Science Skin & Coat and Harrison's Booster and Sunshine Factor have been suggested to be used in stressed, sick, and feather-picking birds. The manufacturer suggests not combining both supplements.

STRESS/ADAPTOGENS

A variety of behavioral issues have been described in exotic species under human care.[117] Strategies have included behavioral modification, changes to the animals' habitats, modification of social structures for the animal and cohorts, and the use of medications. Anxiolytics and hormonal treatments remain popular adjunctive therapies despite potential side effects.[117,118] Natural alternative supplements have been used that contain ingredients that increase serotonin levels.[24,119–121] Serotonin inhibits aggressive behavior in various vertebrates, ranging from teleost fish to primates.[122–124]

In reptiles, stress has been associated with increased plasma catecholamines and corticosterone, reduced testosterone, decreased hepatic protein and vitellogenin synthesis, reduced food intake, fewer breeding displays, and other suppressed or detrimental behaviors[44] These markers of stress in reptiles are increased after capture, restraint, handling, excessive cold or heat, chemical or visual exposure to a dominant male, and deprivation of food and water.[44] Several nutrients are depleted during stress in mammals.[44] The use of serotonin, endogenous opiates, and dopamine in the diet may be helpful.[44] In stressed lizards (*Calotes versicolor*), vitamin C has been reported to decrease over time.[44] Trials of the herbs chamomile (*Matricaria recutita*), echinacea (*Echinacea* spp), ginko (*Ginko biloba*), ginseng (*Panax ginseng*), kava kava (*Piper methysticum*), and valerian (*Valeriana officinalis*) have been reported in more than 20 species with no untoward effects.[44]

In avian species, behavioral problems such as feather picking can be analogous to compulsive grooming disorders in other species.[125] Therefore, similar neurochemical mechanisms may exist that could result in comparable responses to pharmacologic agents.[125] Some cases of obsessive-compulsive disorder and trichotillomania (hair pulling) respond to serotonergic medications, providing evidence that serotonin dysfunction is involved in mediating these behaviors.[125] Serotonergic agents, such as clomipramine, were used successfully to improve feather picking for a 3-week and 6-week trial compared with a placebo group.[125]

Eleven marine institutions using a serotonin supplement completed a survey evaluating the beneficial use for behavior modification. Information on 9 sea lions and 12 dolphins was analyzed.[124] Behaviors before supplementation included 43% of animals displaying interspecies aggression, 19% self-injurious rubbing behavior, 14% human-directed aggression, and 29% fear and/or anxiety associated with social incompatibility or environmental factors.[124] Most animals (67%) showed improvement as measured by a decrease in negative behavioral signs, with 24% showing a complete resolution of behavioral problems.[124] Only 9% of animals failed to show any improvement.[124] No behavioral, physical, or biochemical side effects were reported for any of the animals in the survey.[124] Serotonin-containing supplements may be an effective alternative for aberrant behavioral conditions in mammals and other exotic pets under human care. Other aquatic veterinarians have reported successful use of this supplement to decrease natural, wild sexual behavior in dolphins, sea turtles, and fish.

SUMMARY

By complementing traditional medicine with holistic and alternative nutrition and supplements, the overall health and wellness of exotic pets can be enhanced and balanced. Hippocrates had a strong belief in the power of the body's immune system, stating that, "Our natures are the physicians of ourselves."[126] Further research is needed for understanding the strengths and uses of supplements in exotic species. Caution should always be taken when supplementing pregnant or immature animals. Scientific evidence is increasing in the use of supplements as an adjunctive therapy to conventional medicine. Going back to the animals' origin and roots bring clinicians closer to nature and its healing powers.

ACKNOWLEDGMENTS

The authors acknowledge Dr T. McCalla for her help with editing this article. We also give special thanks to J. Fava and K. Bockhorn for help with editing and formatting charts and references.

REFERENCES

1. Lummis D. Fish, birds, reptiles, and small animals: critical components of the U.S. pet market. Pet Product News International 2013;4. Available at: http://mydigitalpublication.com/publication/?i=148349&p=4. Accessed January 10, 2014.
2. Brown LP. State of the pet supplement industry. 2012. Available at: http://www.nutraceuticalsworld.com/issues/2012-03/view_features/state-of-the-pet-supplement-industry/. Accessed January 10, 2014.
3. Attardo C, Sartori F. Pharmacologically active plant metabolites as survival strategy products. Boll Chim Farm 2003;142:54–65.
4. Larkins N, Wynn S. Pharmacognosy: phytomedicines and their mechanisms. Vet Clin North Am Small Anim Pract 2004;34(1):291–327.
5. Shrivastava R, Apoorva K, Shweta A. Zoopharmacognosy (Animal Self Medication): a review. Int J Basic Appl Physiol 2011;2(5):1510–2.
6. Kang BT, Jung DI, Yoo JH, et al. A high fiber diet responsive case in a poodle dog with long-term plant eating behavior. J Vet Med Sci 2007;69(7):779–82.

7. Smolker R, Richards A, Connor R, et al. Sponge carrying by dolphins (Delphinidae, *Tursiops* sp.): a foraging specialization involving tool use? Ethology 1997; 103:454–65.

8. Meylan A. Spongivory in hawksbill turtles: a diet of glass. Science 1988; 239(4838):393–5.

9. National Center for Complementary and Alternative Medicine. Complementary, alternative, or integrative health: what's in a name? Available at: http://nccam. nih.gov/health/whatiscam. Accessed January 10, 2014.

10. Pappas S, Perlman A. Complementary and alternative medicine. The importance of doctor-patient communication. Med Clin North Am 2002;86(1):1–10.

11. Kidd JR. Alternative medicines for the geriatric veterinary patient. Vet Clin North Am Small Anim Pract 2012;42(4):809–22.

12. Halici M, Imik H, Koç M, et al. Effects of α-lipoic acid, vitamin E and C upon the heat stress in Japanese quails. J Anim Physiol Anim Nutr (Berl) 2012;96(3): 408–15.

13. Carpenter J. Exotics animal formulary. 4th edition. St Louis (MO): Elsevier Saunders; 2013.

14. Pollock C, Carpenter JW, Antinoff N. Birds. In: Carpenter JW, editor. Exotic animal formulary. 3rd edition. St Louis (MO): Elsevier Saunders; 2005. p. 133–344.

15. Orosz SE. Common herbs and their use in avian practice. San Antonio (TX): Association of Avian Veterinarians; 2006.

16. Johnston H, Barron H, Gottdenker N, et al. Plasma antioxidant levels in eastern screech owls (Megascops asio) after supplementation. New Orleans (LA): Association of Avian Veterinarians, in press.

17. Delk KW, Mejia-Fava JC, Jimenez DA, et al. Diagnostic imaging of peripheral vestibular disease in a chinese goose (Anser cygnoides). J Am Vet Med Assoc 2014;28(1):31–7.

18. Thompson R, Wolf T, Rasmussen J. Aspergillosis in African Penguins (*Spheniscus demersus*): understanding diagnostic criteria, treatment, and phophyaxis. Sausalito (CA): International Association of Aquatic Animal Medicine; 2013.

19. Divers SJ, Cooper JE. Hepatic lipidosis. In: Mader DR, editor. Reptile medicine and surgery. St Louis (MO): Saunders Elsevier; 2006. p. 806–12.

20. Ahlstrom RT, Wolf T, Peterson D, et al. Alternative treatment options for managing hepatic lipidosis in an Atlantic Ridley sea turtle (*Lepidocheyls Kempii*). Atlanta (GA): International Association of Aquatic Animal Medicine; 2012.

21. Crow GL. Goiter in elasmobranchs. In: Smith M, Warmolts D, Thoney D, et al, editors. The elasmobranch husbandry manual: captive care of sharks, rays and relatives. Colombus (OH): Biological Survery; 2004. p. 441–6.

22. Rodriguez M, Mejia J, Blanchard M, et al. Pilot Study: the affects of Natramune™ (PDS-2865®) a new immunostimulator supplement on different cetacean species; *Tursiops truncatus, Lagenorhynchus obliquidens*, and *Orcinus orca*. Orlando (FL): International Association of Aquatic Animal Medicine; 2007.

23. Rodriguez M, Mejia J, Blanchard M, et al. Natramune™ (PDS-2865®) an immunostimulator supplement in cetaceans. Pomezia (IT): International Association of Aquatic Animal Medicine; 2008.

24. Doescher B, Mejia-Fava J, Colitz C, et al. Treatment of recurrent chronic ulcerative dermatitis in a bottlenose dolphin (*Tursiops Truncatus*). Las Vegas (NV): International Association of Aquatic Animal Medicine; 2011.

25. Mejia-Fava J, Colitz CM, Don Z, et al. Alpha lipoic acid, a powerful and unique antioxidant: preliminary results following administration of ALA to pinnipeds. Las Vegas (NV): International Association of Aquatic Animal Medicine; 2011.

26. Orosz SE. Application of nutritional supplements and herbs in avian practice. Providence (RI): Association of Avian Veterinarians; 2007.
27. US Food and Drug Administration. Available at: http://www.fda.gov/food/dietarysupplements. Accessed January 10, 2014.
28. Newmaster SG, Grguric M, Shanmughanandhan D, et al. DNA barcoding defects contamination and substitution in North American herbal products. BMC Med 2013;11(222):1–13.
29. Ross CA. Vitamin A. In: Coates PM, Betz JM, Blackman MR, et al, editors. Encyclopedia of dietary supplements. 2nd edition. London; New York: Informa Healthcare; 2010. p. 778–91.
30. Koutsos EA, Tell LA, Woods LW, et al. Adult cockatiels (Nymphicus hollandicus) at maintenance are more sensitive to diets containing excess vitamin A than to vitamin A-deficient diets. J Nutr 2003;133(6):1898–902.
31. Brubacher GB, Weiser H. The vitamin A activity of beta-carotene. Int J Vitam Nutr Res 1985;55(1):5–15.
32. Hickenbottom SJ. Dual isotope test for assessing beta-carotene cleavage to Vitamin A in humans. Eur J Nutr 2002;41(4):141–7.
33. Stahl S. Hypovitaminosis A. In: Mayer J, Donnelly TM, editors. Clinical veterinary advisor birds and exotic pets. St Louis (MO): Elsevier Saunders; 2013. p. 110–2.
34. Anderson PA, Huber DR, Berzins IK. Correlations of capture, transport, and nutrition in sandtiger sharks, Carcharias Taurus, in public aquaria. J Zoo Wildl Med 2012;43(4):750–8.
35. Moleiro de López MG, Herrera de Rincón MI. Hypervitaminosis C and orthodontic movement. A histological study in the guinea pig periodontium. Acta Odontol Venez 1983;21(11):111–27.
36. Holick MF, Chen TC, Lu Z, et al. Vitamin D and skin physiology: a D-lightful story. J Bone Miner Res 2007;22:V28–33.
37. Tripkovic L, Lambert H, Smith CP, et al. Comparison of vitamin D2 and vitamin D3 supplementation in raising serum 25-dehydroxyvitamin D status: a systemic review and meta-analysis. Am J Clin Nutr 2012;95(6):1357–64.
38. Stahl S. Nutritional secondary hyperparathyroidism. In: Mayer J, Donnelly TM, editors. Clinical veterinary advisor birds and exotic pets. St Louis (MO): Elsevier Saunders; 2013. p. 121–5.
39. Haroon M, FitzGerald O. Vitamin and its emerging role immunopathology. Clin Rheumatol 2012;31:199–202.
40. Fujita A. Thiaminase. In: Nord FF, editor. Advances in enzymology, vol. 15. New York: Interscience; 1954. p. 389–421.
41. Croft LA, Gearhart SA, Heym K, et al. Thiamine deficiency in a collection of pacific harbor seals (Phoca vitulina). Las Vegas (NV): International Association of Aquatic Animal Medicine; 2011.
42. Geraci JR. Experimental thiamine deficiency in captive harp seals, phoca groenlandica, induced by eating herring, clupea harengus, and smelts, osmerus, mordax. Can J Zool 1972;50:179–95.
43. Geraci JR. Thiamine deficiency in seals and recommendations for its prevention. J Am Vet Med Assoc 1974;165:801–3.
44. Donoghue S. Nutrition. In: Mader DR, editor. Reptile medicine and surgery. 2nd edition. St Louis (MO): Elsevier Saunders; 2006. p. 289–90.
45. Worthy GA. Nutrition and energentics. In: Dierauf LA, Gulland FM, editors. CRC handbook of marine mammal medicine. 2nd edition. Boca Raton (FL): CRC Press LLC; 2001. p. 811–27.

46. Dierenfield E, Katz N, et al. Retinol and alpha-tocopherol concentrations in whole fish commonly fed in zoos and aquariums. Zoo Biol 1991;10:119–25.
47. Mejia-Fava J, Bossart GD, Hoopes L, et al. Nutritional analysis of frozen Canadian Capelin (*Mallotus villosus*), Atlantic Herring (*Clupea harengus*), and Candian Lake Smelt (*Osmerus mordax*) over a 9 month period of frozen storage. Gold Coast (AU): International Association of Aquatic Animal Medicine; 2014.
48. Maffei Facino R, Carini M, Aldini G, et al. Sparing effect of procyanidins from *Vitis vinifera* on vitamin E: in vitro studies. Planta Med 1998;64(4):343–7.
49. Carini M, Maffei Facino R, Aldini G, et al. The protection of polyunsaturated fatty acids in micellar systems against UVB-induced photo-oxidation by procyanidins from *Vitis vinifera L*., and the protective synergy with vitamin E. Int J Cosmet Sci 1998;20(4):203–15.
50. Bagchi D, Garg A, Krohn RL, et al. Oxygen free radical scavenging abilities of vitamins C and E, and a grape seed proanthocyanidin extract in vitro. Res Commun Mol Pathol Pharmacol 1997;95(2):179–89.
51. Schoemaker NJ, Lumeij JT, Dorrestein GM, et al. Nutrion-related problems in pet birds]. Bird-goiter paper. Tijdschr Diergeneeskd 1999;124(2):39–43 [in Dutch].
52. Topper MJ, McManamon R, Thorstad CL. Colloid goiter in an eastern diamondback rattlesnake (*Crotalus adamanteus*). Vet Pathol 1994;31:380–2.
53. Morris AL, Stremme DW, Sheppard BJ, et al. The onset of Goiter in several species of sharks following the addition of ozone to a touch pool. J Zoo Wildl Med 2012;43(3):621–4.
54. Lall SP. The minerals. In: Halver JE, editor. Fish nutrition A. San Diego (CA): Academic Press Inc; 1989. p. 219–57.
55. Gómez-Jacinto V, Arias-Borrego A, Garcia-Barrera T, et al. Iodine speciation in iodine-enriched microalgae *Chlorella vulgaris*. Pure Appl Chem 2010;82(2): 473–81.
56. Mazo VK, Gmoshinshïĭ IV, Zilova IS. Microalgae Spirulina in human nutrition. Vopr Pitan 2004;73(1):45–53.
57. Khachik F, de Moura FF, Zhao DY, et al. Transformations of selected carotenoids in plasma, liver, and ocular tissues of humans and in nonhuman primate animal models. Invest Ophthalmol Vis Sci 2002;43:3383–92.
58. Yeum KJ, Taylor A, Tang G, et al. Measurement of carotenoids, retinoids, and tocopherols in human lenses. Invest Ophthalmol Vis Sci 1995;36:2756–61.
59. Krinsky NI. Possible biological mechanisms for a protective role of xanthophylls. J Nutr 2002;132:540S–2S.
60. Snodderly DM, Auran JD, Delori FC. The macular pigment. II. Spatial distribution in primate retinas. Invest Ophthalmol Vis Sci 1984;25:674–85.
61. Rapp LM, Maple SS, Choi JH. Lutein and zeaxanthin concentrations in rod outer segment membranes from perifoveal and peripheral human retina. Invest Ophthalmol Vis Sci 2000;41:1200–9.
62. Wang Y, Connor SL, Wang W, et al. The selective retention of lutein, meso-zeaxanthin and zeaxanthin in the retina of chicks fed a xanthophyll-free diet. Exp Eye Res 2007;84:591–8.
63. Koutsos EA, Schmitt T, Colitz CM, et al. Absorption and ocular deposition of dietary lutein in marine mammals. Zoo Biol 2013;32:316–23.
64. Mejia-Fava J, Barron H, Blas-Machodo U, et al. High infertility, perinatal morbidity and mortality, and mucocutaneous lesion in Captive Green Sea Turtles(Chelonia Mydas) associated with carotenoid deficiency. Vancouver (Canada): International Association of Aquatic Animal Medicine; 2010.

65. Jin XH, Ohgami K, Shiratory K, et al. Inhibitory effects of lutein on endotoxin-induced uveitis in Lewis rats. Invest Ophthalmol Vis Sci 2006;47:2562–8.
66. Gupta SK, Trivedi D, Srivastava S, et al. Lycopene attenuates oxidative stress induced experimental cataract development: an in vitro and in vivo study. Nutrition 2003;19:794–9.
67. Durukan AH, Everklioglu C, Hurmeric V, et al. Ingestion of IH636 grape seed proanthocyanidin extract to prevent selenite-induced oxidative stress in experimental cataract. J Cataract Refract Surg 2006;32:1041–5.
68. Zhang B, Safa R, Rusciano D, et al. Epigallocatechin gallate, an active ingredient from green tea, attenuates damaging influences to the retina caused by ischemia/reperfusion. Brain Res 2007;1159:40–53.
69. Falsini B, Maranngoni D, Salgarello T, et al. Effect of epigallocatechin-gallate on inner retinal function in ocular hypertension and glaucoma: a short-term study by pattern electroretinogram. Graefes Arch Clin Exp Ophthalmol 2009;247:1223–33.
70. Mandel SA, Avramovich-Tirosh Y, Reznichenko L, et al. Multifunctional activities of green tea catechins in neuroprotection. Modulation of cell survival genes, iron-dependent oxidatives stress and PKC signaling pathway. Neurosignals 2005;14:46–60.
71. Zhang B, Osborn NN. Oxidative-induced retinal degeneration is attenuated by epgallocatechin gallate. Brain Res 2006;1124:176–87.
72. Chu KO, Chan KP, Wang CC, et al. Green tea catechins and their oxidation protection in the rat eye. J Agric Food Chem 2010;58:1523–34.
73. Gupta SK, Halder N, Srivastava S, et al. Green tea (Camellia sinensis) protects against selenite-induced oxidative stress in experimental cataractogenesis. Ophthalmic Res 2002;34:258–63.
74. Manach C, Morand C, Crespy V, et al. Quercetin is recovered in human plasma as conjugated derivatives which retain antioxidant properties. FEBS Lett 1998;426:331–6.
75. Cornish KM, Williamson G, Sanderson J. Quercetin metabolism in the lens: role in inhibition of hydrogen peroxide induced cataract. Free Radic Biol Med 2002;33:63–70.
76. Neuringer M, Anderson GJ, Connor WE. The essentiality of N-3 fatty acids for the development and function of the retina and brain. Annu Rev Nutr 1988;8:517–41.
77. Tinoco J. Dietary requirements and functions of alpha-linolenic acid in animals. Prog Lipid Res 1982;21:1–45.
78. Chucair AJ, Rotstein NP, SanGiovanni JP, et al. Lutein and zeaxanthin protect photoreceptors from apoptosis induced by oxidatives stress: relation with docosahexaenoic acid. Invest Ophthalmol Vis Sci 2007;48:5168–77.
79. Jocelyn PC. Thiols and disulfides in animal tissues. Biochemistry of the SH groups. London: Academic Press; 1972.
80. Smith AR, Shenvi SV, Widlansky M, et al. Lipoic acid as a potential therapy for chronic diseases associated with oxidative stress. Curr Med Chem 2004;11:1135–46.
81. Peinado J, Sies H, Akerboom TP. Hepatic lipoate uptake. Arch Biochem Biophys 1989;273:389–95.
82. Maitra I, Serbinova E, Trischler H, et al. Alpha-lipoic acid prevents buthionine sulfoximine-induced cataract formation in newborn rats. Free Radic Biol Med 1995;18:823–9.

83. Miranda M, Arnal E, Ahuja S, et al. Antioxidants rescue photoreceptors in rd1 mice: Relationship with thiol metabolism. Free Radic Biol Med 2010; 48:216–22.
84. Holan KM. Feline hepatic lipidosis. In: Kirk RW, editor. Current veterinary therapy XIV. St Louis (MO): Saunders Elsevier; 2009. p. 570–5.
85. Mcarthur S. Problem-solving approach to common diseases of terrestrial and semi-aquatic chelonians. In: Mcarthur S, Wilkenson R, Meyer J, editors. Medicine and surgery of tortoises and turtles. Oxford (United Kingdom): Blackwell; 2004. p. 333–5.
86. Beaufrère H, Taylor M. Hepatic lipidosis. In: Mayer J, Donnelly TM, editors. Clinical veterinary advisor birds and exotic pets. St Louis (MO): Elsevier Saunders; 2013. p. 194–7.
87. Roudybush TE. Psittacine nutrition. Vet Clin North Am Exot Anim Pract 1999; 2(1):111–25.
88. Shay KP, Moreau RF, Smith EJ, et al. Alpha-lipoic acid as a dietary supplement: molecular mechanisms and therapeutic potential. Biochim Biophys Acta 2009; 1790(10):1149–60.
89. Hill AS, Werner JA, Rogers QR, et al. Lipoic acid is 10 times more toxic in cats than reported in humans, dogs or rats. J Anim Physiol Anim Nutr (Berl) 2004; 88(3-4):150–6.
90. Shih JC. Atherosclerosis in Japanese quail and the effect of lipoic acid. Fed Proc 1983;42(8):2494–7.
91. Bottiglieri T. Folate, vitamin B12, and S-adenosylnethionine. Psychiatr Clin North Am 2013;36(1):1–13.
92. Center SA. Metabolic, antioxidant, nutraceutical, probiotic, and herbal therapies relating to the management of hepatobiliary disorders. Vet Clin North Am Small Anim Pract 2004;34:67–172.
93. Thomson MA, Baur BA, Loehrer LL, et al. Dietary supplement S-adenosyl-L-methionine (AdoMet) effects on plasma homocysteine levels in healthy human subjects: a double-blind, placebo-controlled, randomized clinical trial. J Altern Complement Med 2009;15(5):523–9.
94. Kidd PM. Phosphatidylcholine: a superior protectant against liver damage. Altern Med Rev 1999;4(1):258–74.
95. Nieminen P, Mustonen AM, Kärjä V, et al. Fatty acid composition and development of hepatic lipidosis during food deprivation-mustelids as a potential animal model for liver steatosis. Exp Biol Med (Maywood) 2009;243(9):278–86.
96. Patterson W, Wall R, Fitzgerald GF, et al. Health implications of high dietary omega-6 polyunsaturated fatty acids. J Nutr Metab 2012;2012:539426.
97. Kulza M, Adamska K, Seńczuk-Przybyłowska M, et al. Artichoke-herbal drug. Przegl 2012;69(10):1122–6.
98. Grizzle J, Hadley TL, Rotstein DS, et al. Effects of dietary milk thistle on blood parameters, liver pathology, and hepatobiliary scintigraphy in white carneaux pigeons (Columba livia) challenged with B1 aflatoxin. J Avian Med Surg 2009; 23(2):114–24.
99. Colle D, Arantes LP, Gubert P, et al. Antioxidant properties of *Taraxacum officinale* leaf extract are involved in the protective effect against hepatotoxicity induced by acetaminophen in mice. J Med Food 2012;5(6):549–56.
100. Davaatseren M, Hur HJ, Yang HJ, et al. Dandelion leaf extract protects against liver injury induced by methionine- and choline-deficient diet in mice. J Med Food 2013;16(1):26–33.

101. Chavoustie S, Perez P, Fletcher M, et al. Pilot Study: effect of PDS-2865 on natural killer cell cytoxicity. Journal on Nutraceuticals and Nutrition 2003;6(2): 39–42.
102. Weeks BS, Perez P. The hemicelluloses preparation Natramune (PDS-2865™) increases macrophage phagocytosis and nitric oxide production and increases circulating human lymphocytes levels. Med Sci Monit 2009;15(2):43–6.
103. Weeks BS, Lee SW, Perez P, et al. Natramune and PureWay-C reduce xenobiotic- induced human T-cell alpha5beta1 integrin-mediated adhesion to fibronectin. Med Sci Monit 2008;14(12):279–85.
104. Kelly GS. Large arabinogalactan: clinical relevance of a novel immune-enhancing polysaccharide. Altern Med Rev 1999;4(2):96–103.
105. Jiang W, Zhu Z, McGinley JN, et al. Identification of a molecular underlying inhibition of mammary carcinoma growth by dietary N-3 fatty acids. Cancer Res 2012;72(15):3795–806.
106. Schaffer HK. Essential fatty acids and eicosanoids in cutaneous inflammation. Int J Dermatol 1989;28(5):281–90.
107. Kelly GS. Squalene and its potential clinical uses. Altern Med Rev 1999;4(1): 29–36.
108. Gazim ZC, Rezende CM, Fraga SR, et al. Antifungal activity of the essential oil from *Calendula officinalis L.* (asteraceae) growing in Brazil. Braz J Microbiol 2008;39(1):61–3.
109. Kumari AM, Devi PU, Sucharitha A. Differential effect of lipoxygenase on aflatoxin production by *Aspergillus spp.* International Journal of Plant Pathology 2011;4:153–64.
110. Gross NT, Hultenby K, Mengarelli S, et al. Lipid peroxidation by alveolar macrophages challenged with *Cryptococcus neoformans, Candida albicans, or Aspergillus fumigatus.* Med Mycol 2000;38(6):443–9.
111. McBride PT, Clark L, Kruger GG. Evaluation of triacontanol-containing compunds as anti-inflammatory agents using guinea pig models. J Invest Dermatol 1987;89(4):380–3.
112. Ramanarayan K, Bhat A, Shripathi V, et al. Triacontanol inhibits both enzymatic and nonenzymatic lipid peroxidation. Phytochemistry 2000;55:59–66. Elsevier Science Ltd.
113. Marcelletti JF, Lusso P, Katz DH. N-Docosanol inhibits in vitro replication of HIV and other retroviruses. AIDS Res Hum Retroviruses 1996;12:71–4.
114. Lawrence R, Tripathi P, Jeyakumar E. Isolation, purification and evaluation of antibacterial agents from Aloe vera. Braz J Microbiol 2009;40(4):906–15.
115. Boateng J, Verghese M, Chawan CB, et al. Red palm oil suppresses the formation of azoxymethane (AOM) induced aberrant crypt (ACF) in Fisher 344 male rats. Food Chem Toxicol 2006;44(10):1667–73.
116. Szucs G, Bester DJ, Kupai K, et al. Dietary red palm oil supplementation decreases infarct size in cholesterol fed rats. Lipids Health Dis 2011;10:103.
117. Crowell-Davis SL, Murray T. Veterinary psychopharmacology. Ames (IA): Blackwell Publishing; 2006.
118. Manire CA. The use of megestrol acetate in atlantic bottlenose dolphins. Vancouver (Canada): International Association of Aquatic Animal Medicine; 2010.
119. Crupi R, Mazzon E, Marino A, et al. Hypericum perforatum treatment: effect on behaviour and neurogenesis in a chronic stress model in mice. BMC Complement Altern Med 2011;11:7.
120. Fiebich BL, Knörle R, Appel K, et al. Pharmacological studies in an herbal drug combination of St. John's Wort (*Hypericum perforatum*) and passion flower

(*Passiflora incarnata*): in vitro and in vivo evidence of synergy between Hypericum and Passiflora in antidepressant pharmacological models. Fitoterapia 2010;82:474–80.

121. Kimura Y, Sumiyoshi M. Effects of various Eleutherococcus senticosus cortex on swimming time, natural killer activity and corticosterone level in forced swimming stressed mice. J Ethnopharmacol 2004;95:447–53.

122. Edwards DH, Kravitz EA. Serotonin, social status and aggression. Curr Opin Neurobiol 1997;7:812–9.

123. Wingerg S, Øverli Ø, Lepage O. Suppression of aggression in rainbow trout (*Oncorhynchus mykiss*) by dietary L-tryptophan. J Exp Biol 2001;204:3867–76.

124. Doescher BM, Mejia-Fava J, Pawloski J. Serenin Vet™, a natural alternative supplement, used as an adjunct for marine mammal behavior modification. Atlanta (GA): International Association of Aquatic Animal Medicine; 2012.

125. Seibert LM, Crowell-Davis SL, Wilson HG, et al. Placebo-controlled clomipramine trial for the treatment of feather picking disorder in cockatoos. J Am Anim Hosp Assoc 2004;40:261–9.

126. Bellavite P, Andrioli G, Lussignoli S, et al. A scientific reappraisal of the 'principal of similarity'. Med Hypotheses 1997;49(3):203–12.

Index

Note: Page numbers of article titles are in **boldface** type.

A

Abscesses, aural, in reptiles, 378
    dental, in rabbits, 488
Acceptance of food. See *Behavioral considerations.*
Acetate energy, in macropods, 429–430
Acid base correction, for rabbits, with hepatic lipidosis, 492
      with urolithiasis, 491
Acid detergent fraction (ADF), 357
Adaptogens, as supplements, 517–518
Aeromonas hydrophila, for aquatic animals, 336
Aflatoxins, in food, 341, 411
Alfalfa, for chinchillas and guinea pigs, 472, 476
    for marsupials, 432
    for rabbits, 499–500
Algae, for aquatic animal nutrition, 336, 344
Alpha lipoic acid (ALA), for fish, 508
    for liver support, 513–514
    for reptiles, 508
    ocular effects of, 513
Alternative medicine, supplements vs., 505
American Association of Feed Control Officials (AAFCO), 338
Amino acids, essential, for aquatic animals, 334
      for avians, 401–402, 408–409
      for ferrets, 451–452, 456
      for reptiles, 508
      for rodent, 476–477
    in feeder insects, for amphibians, 357
Ammonia, excretion of, in aquatic animals, 338–339
    production of, in macropods, 430–431
Amphibian nutrition, **347–367**
    diet components of, 350–351
    digestibility challenges with, 356, 359–360
    gastrointestinal anatomy and, 348–350
      in adults, 348–350
      in larvae, 348
    insects in, nutrient composition of, 351–356
      nutritive value of, 347–348
        optimizing, 360–362
    introduction to, 347–348
    key points of, 347
    nutrient bioavailability of, 357, 359–360
    nutrient components/requirements for, 356–359

Vet Clin Exot Anim 17 (2014) 527–566
http://dx.doi.org/10.1016/S1094-9194(14)00050-4
1094-9194/14/$ – see front matter © 2014 Elsevier Inc. All rights reserved.

vetexotic.theclinics.com

Moving?

Make sure your subscription moves with you!

To notify us of your new address, find your **Clinics Account Number** (located on your mailing label above your name), and contact customer service at:

Email: journalscustomerservice-usa@elsevier.com

800-654-2452 (subscribers in the U.S. & Canada)
314-447-8871 (subscribers outside of the U.S. & Canada)

Fax number: 314-447-8029

Elsevier Health Sciences Division
Subscription Customer Service
3251 Riverport Lane
Maryland Heights, MO 63043

*To ensure uninterrupted delivery of your subscription, please notify us at least 4 weeks in advance of move.

Printed and bound by CPI Group (UK) Ltd, Croydon, CR0 4YY

03/10/2024

01040465-0006